Bottom Line's
Hushed-Up 100

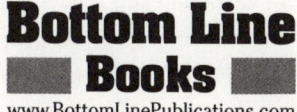

Bottom Line Books
www.BottomLinePublications.com

Copyright © 2014 by Boardroom® Inc.

All rights reserved. No part of this publication may be reproduced, scanned, distributed or transmitted in any form, by any means, electronic or mechanical, without permission in writing from the publisher.

First printing

Bottom Line Books® publishes the advice of expert authorities in many fields. These opinions may at times conflict as there are often different approaches to solving problems. The use of this material is no substitute for health, legal, accounting or other professional services. Consult competent professionals for answers to your specific questions.

Telephone numbers, addresses, prices, offers and Web sites listed in this book are accurate at the time of publication, but they are subject to frequent change.

Bottom Line Books® is a registered trademark of
Boardroom® Inc.
281 Tresser Boulevard, Stamford, CT 06901

www.bottomlinepublications.com

Bottom Line Books® is an imprint of Boardroom® Inc., publisher of print periodicals, e-letters and books. We are dedicated to bringing you the best information from the most knowledgeable sources in the world. Our goal is to help you gain greater wealth, better health, more wisdom, extra time and increased happiness.

Printed in the United States of America

HBT/am

Contents

#1	The Cholesterol Study You Never Saw	1
#2	Clean Clogged Arteries for Free	2
#3	Could This B Vitamin Boost Your Hearing?	4
#4	The New Anticancer Formula	5
#5	Alternatives for Uncomfortable Sleep Apnea Treatments	6
#6	The Accidental Cure for High Blood Pressure	8
#7	Pop a Purple Potato to Lower Blood Pressure	9
#8	More Than 80% of Blood Pressure Readings Are Wrong	9
#9	FDA Approves Drug That Shows Promise for Certain Breast Cancers	10
#10	Pain Killer Lowers Breast Cancer Recurrence	11
#11	Eat Dark Meat for a Healthier Heart	11
#12	The Instant Migraine Eraser	12
#13	Injection Helps Cancer Patients Live Pain Free	13
#14	Keep Your Hair During Chemo	13
#15	Reduce Your Breast Cancer Risk by 23%	14
#16	Fish Oil Works as Well as Drugs to Treat Depression	15
#17	Pumpkin Seeds Boost Mood	16
#18	Fruit Conquers Jet Lag	16
#19	Vitamin D Eases Breast Cancer Drug Pain	16
#20	Drinks That Melt Your Teeth	17
#21	What's Killing Older Americans?	18
#22	Test Predicts Lung Cancer Survival	18
#23	The Covered-Up Cause of IBS	19
#24	Best Ways to Avoid Painful Diverticulitis	19
#25	Citrus Supplement Helps Stop Cancer From Spreading	20
#26	Raise Your IQ Nine Points in 10 Minutes	22
#27	Hope for Patients with Inoperable Tumors	23
#28	The Nose Spray That "Eats Away" Alzheimer's Plaques	24
#29	Some Drugs No Better Than Placebo for Alzheimer's Patients	25
#30	"Old Age" Symptoms Could Really Be a Vitamin Deficiency	26
#31	How Nicotine Patches May Help Get Your Memory Back	28
#32	The "Clothing Cure" for Glaucoma	29
#33	Top Antihistamine Doesn't Work!	30
#34	Protect the Family from the Flu— No Vaccine Needed	31
#35	Never Use a Spoon to Measure Meds	32
#36	Don't Drink the Water	33
#37	Deadly Virus Found in Florida	35
#38	Cold Sores May Be Linked to Alzheimer's Disease	35
#39	A New Treatment May Eliminate Tinnitus	35
#40	Beans Lower Blood Sugar	35
#41	Yes, You Can Prevent Diabetes Complications	36

#	Title	Page
#42	Diabetic Kidney Disease Supplement May Help	38
#43	Topical Gel Beats Bladder Problems	39
#44	Newer Blood Thinner Dangerous for Trauma Patients	39
#45	The 15-Minute Heart Cure	40
#46	Breakthrough! First New Lupus Drug in More Than 50 Years	42
#47	Chest Pains—What They Mean… What to Do	43
#48	Standard Heart Tests Fail to Show True Risks	44
#49	Up to 80% of Heart Failure Cases Could Be Prevented	46
#50	Say Good-Bye to Your Diabetes Medication	48
#51	The "Cooking Oil Cure" for High Blood Pressure	49
#52	How Brain Scientist Jill Bolte Taylor Came Back from a Stroke	50
#53	Can Diet Soda Boost Your Stroke Risk?	52
#54	How to Lose 12 Pounds…in Just 17 Days	53
#55	Are You Taking a Drug That Isn't FDA Approved for Your Illness?	54
#56	Prozac Speeds Stroke Recovery	55
#57	Pulverize Precancerous Prostate Cells	57
#58	Major Breakthrough in Brain Health	59
#59	Listen Up! These Vitamins Can Prevent Hearing Loss	61
#60	Cancer-Free in a Week	62
#61	Strawberries Join the Fight Against Cancer	63
#62	The Ultimate Lab Test: Dogs That Sniff Out Colon Cancer	64
#63	Melatonin: New Help for Heartburn	66
#64	New Treatment for Cataracts	67
#65	Early Morning Colonoscopies Find 27% More Polyps	67
#66	The Truth About Life After Prostate Cancer	67
#67	Why I Love Lasers to Zap Fat	70
#68	The Ultimate Natural Weight-Loss Aid	71
#69	The Blood Pressure Pill That's Great for Your Bones	72
#70	Ginger Slows Tumor Growth by 56%	73
#71	Seek Support to Survive Diabetes	74
#72	Drop Pounds and Blood Sugar— with Vinegar	75
#73	The "Coffee Cure" for High Blood Sugar	75
#74	Diabetes Reversed!	76
#75	Attention Women: Diabetes Linked to Irregular Heartbeat Risk	77
#76	Pain Relievers Are Linked to Erectile Dysfunction	77
#77	How to Firm Up Man Breasts	77
#78	The Secret Cause of Asthma?	77
#79	The Secret Recipe for Hair Growth	78
#80	Oregano for Arthritis	79
#81	Are Pain Medications Sapping Your Sex Life?	80
#82	The Truth About Garlic—Health Claims That You Can Trust	80
#83	You May Not Need a Knee Replacement	82
#84	Mike's Miracle Vision Cure	83
#85	Natural Painkiller Works Better Than Morphine	84
#86	DMSO—Rub On Quick Pain Relief	85
#87	Psoriasis Stopped for Eight Out of 10 Patients	86
#88	How to Avoid the NEW Medicare Scam	87
#89	FDA OKs Valve That Does Not Require Open Heart Surgery	89
#90	New Treatment for Severe Migraines	91
#91	Grow Your Own "New" Heart	90
#92	Aspirin Works as Well as Warfarin for Heart Failure Patients	92
#93	Love: Nature's Powerful Painkiller?	93
#94	SHINE Helps Fibromyalgia	94
#95	Contamination Alert!	94
#96	Don't Chop Those Carrots!	94
#97	Warning: We're No Longer Sweet on Agave	95
#98	Natural Relief for Fibrocystic Breasts	95
#99	Ways to Fight Lingering Shingles Pain	96
#100	Rise in Some Head and Neck Cancers Tied to Sexual Activity	97

Bottom Line's Hushed-Up 100

REPORT #1
The Cholesterol Study You Never Saw

Statins really do lower cholesterol, but that doesn't automatically mean a lower risk of heart problems or death compared with conventional therapy to lower blood fat, say researchers.

Still, experts say the results don't undermine the broad utility of statins, which are among the most widely prescribed drugs on the planet. Rather, the study suggests doctors need to do a better job of keeping patients on the medications if they expect the same performance produced by rigorous clinical trials.

This is not a blemish on statins, according to Richard C. Pasternak, MD, a Harvard University cardiologist. "It's more a blemish on our ability to maintain best practice," he says.

STATINS' STATUS

In previous studies, statins have led to marked reductions in total cholesterol and low-density lipoprotein (LDL), or the "bad," form of blood fat. However, those trials have been in tightly controlled settings that don't necessarily reflect the real world. They also typically involved people with high or extremely high cholesterol.

A recent study involved more than 10,000 people with moderately high cholesterol, high blood pressure under control with medication and at least one risk factor for heart disease, such as type 2 diabetes.

Half the patients got *pravastatin* (Pravachol) ...the rest received the usual advice to make lifestyle changes, such as a low-fat diet and exercise. Nearly one-third of those in the latter group switched to pravastatin during the eight-year study.

Richard C. Pasternak, MD, director of preventive cardiology, Massachusetts General Hospital, and associate professor of medicine, Harvard Medical School, Boston.

Barry R. Davis, MD, PhD, director of the ALLHAT Clinical Trials Center, and professor of biometry, University of Texas School of Public Health, Houston.

Joshua S. Benner, PharmD, ScD, formerly director of health economics, Epinomics Research, Alexandria, Virginia.

The Journal of the American Medical Association

After four years, people taking the statin drug saw their total cholesterol drop by approximately twice as much as those in the other group.

However, the gap between the two groups for total cholesterol was less than half the average of eight other large studies comparing statins with other therapies.

The number of deaths in each group was essentially identical, as were the rates of nonfatal heart attacks and deadly artery trouble.

"The [clinical] trials provide a compelling case for statin use, but in the real world, it doesn't appear that patients are getting the full benefit that the trials suggest," says Joshua S. Benner, formerly director of health economics at Epinomics Research, a Virginia–based consulting firm.

STATINS STILL WORK

Barry Davis, MD, PhD, who ran the latest study at the University of Texas Health Science Center in Houston, explains that the benefits of the statin were obscured by patients switching out of the usual care group and into the statin arm of the study. That migration was prompted by the evidence of the drug's ability to prevent cardiovascular deaths made public during the late 1990s. If no one had switched, they probably would have seen a difference in death rates, he says.

You can learn more about statins at The HealthCentral Network at *www.heartinfo.org*.

REPORT #2
Clean Clogged Arteries For Free

Mark A. Stengler, NMD, naturopathic medical doctor and leading authority on the practice of alternative and integrated medicine. Dr. Stengler is author of the *Health Revelations* newsletter, author of *The Natural Physician's Healing Therapies* (Bottom Line Books), founder and medical director of the Stengler Center for Integrative Medicine in Encinitas, California, and adjunct associate clinical professor at the National College of Natural Medicine in Portland, Oregon. *http://markstengler.com*

Amid the clamor created by pharmaceutical companies hyping cholesterol-lowering statin drugs, important information is going unheard.

You need to know: Four natural therapies can protect, and even restore, the health of your arteries—without the dangerous side effects of statin drugs.

These natural substances help to reverse the process of plaque buildup—to dissolve plaque, eliminating the danger it presents. They are available over-the-counter from health-food stores, online and/or from holistic physicians. Unless otherwise noted, they have no serious side effects, can be taken indefinitely and are generally safe for everyone, including people who take statin drugs. *Important...*

• **If you have atherosclerosis or any other cardiovascular condition,** you need to be under a cardiologist's care.

• **If you take blood-thinning medication,** such as aspirin or *warfarin* (Coumadin)—typically given to improve blood flow and prevent blood clots—talk to your doctor before using the natural therapies below, because they could affect your medication dosage.

• **If you are pregnant,** speak to your doctor before taking these or any other supplements or drugs.

• **Discontinue use of these substances 10 to 14 days prior to scheduled surgery** to reduce the risk of excess bleeding. Resume use according to your doctor's instructions (typically 10 days after the procedure).

• **To determine which substance or combination of substances to use,** see "The Right Regimen for You" at the end of this article.

1. TOCOTRIENOLS

Vitamin E is not just one vitamin, but rather a family of eight slightly different molecular structures that function differently in the body. There are two principal categories of vitamin E, called *tocopherols* and *tocotrienols*. Each of these has four subcategories—alpha, beta, gamma and delta.

Some vitamin E supplements contain synthetic alpha-tocopherol. If that's what is in your cupboard—indicated on the label as "dl-alpha-tocopherol"—throw it away now! Synthetic alpha-tocopherol hogs the space on cells' vitamin E receptors (slots into which molecules must fit in order to be used by the body), leaving less room for the more healthful tocopherols you ingest from food or natural supplements (labeled "d-alpha-tocopherol"). Natural tocopherols reduce free radicals, helping to prevent new plaque, but they have not been shown to reduce plaque that is already present. For that, you need tocotrienols.

Tocotrienols are found in rice bran, coconut, barley and wheat germ—but only in small amounts. Supplements with mixed tocopherols/tocotrienols are sold in health-food stores—but they are not the best for reducing plaque.

Better: A tocotrienol-only supplement. I like Allergy Research Group Delta-Fraction Tocotrienols (800-545-9960, *www.allergyresearchgroup.com*), available from holistic doctors. The dosage is 300 milligrams (mg) per day.

2. VITAMIN K

Vitamin K protects against harmful arterial calcification. Forms of vitamin K include *phylloquinone* (K1) and *menaquinone* (K2). Vitamin K1 is abundant in dark green leafy vegetables, such as lettuce, spinach and broccoli. However, vitamin K2 is better absorbed and remains active in the body longer than vitamin K1. Good food sources of vitamin K2 include natto (fermented soybeans) and, to a lesser degree, fermented cheeses (the type with holes, such as Swiss and Jarlsberg), beef liver, chicken and egg yolks.

People taking warfarin are at higher risk for atherosclerosis and osteoporosis (brittle bones) due to the drug's effects on calcification. A study in *Pharmacotherapy* demonstrated the safety and benefit of low-dose vitamin K supplementation in patients taking warfarin. Vitamin K also promotes beneficial bone calcification.

Note: It is vital that a person who takes blood thinners use vitamin K only under the close supervision of a doctor, because the medication dosage may need to be adjusted.

Research suggests that most people get too little vitamin K. I think daily supplementation with 150 to 200 micrograms (mcg) of vitamin K2 is appropriate for all adults—and especially important for those with atherosclerosis. If you take warfarin, the daily dose may be modified, depending on blood tests that indicate how your clotting mechanism interacts with vitamin K. A brand I like is Jarrow Formula's MK-7 (800-726-0886, *www.jarrow.com*).

3. GARLIC EXTRACT

Legend tells us that garlic protects against vampires—but its true power lies in its ability to protect arteries. Most beneficial is *aged garlic extract* (AGE), available in capsule or liquid form. A study from the University of California, Los Angeles, involved 19 cardiac patients who were taking statin drugs and aspirin daily. Participants took either a placebo or 4 milliliters (ml) of a liquid brand called Kyolic AGE for one year.

Findings: Participants who took AGE had about a 66% reduction in new plaque formation compared with those who took a placebo.

Research demonstrates that AGE also can...

•**Reduce LDL cholesterol by up to 12%... total cholesterol by up to 31%...and triglycerides by up to 19%.**

•**Protect against the LDL oxidation that can trigger arterial plaque formation.**

•**Thin the blood.**

•**Lower blood pressure.**

•**Reduce blood levels of homocysteine—**the amino acid that, when elevated, may raise cardiovascular disease risk.

•**Reduce C-reactive protein,** which is a blood marker of inflammation and a risk factor for atherosclerosis.

•**Combat carotid plaque.**

I recommend supplementing daily with AGE.

Dosage: 4 ml to 6 ml of liquid AGE or 400 mg to 600 mg in tablet or capsule form.

4. POMEGRANATE JUICE

Once considered exotic, pomegranate juice now is sold in supermarkets and is a proven boon to arterial health. Israeli researchers verified this in a three-year study of 19 men and women, ages 65 to 75, with severe carotid artery blockage. Ten participants drank 50 ml (about two ounces) per day of 100% pomegranate juice, and nine participants drank a placebo.

Results: Among juice drinkers, plaque thickness decreased by an average of 13% after three months and 35% after one year. This is phenomenal—no drug can come close to reducing plaque like this! Placebo drinkers had a 9% increase in plaque after one year.

Pomegranate juice is loaded with antioxidants called polyphenols, which prevent cholesterol oxidation and improve blood flow.

Note: Choose 100% juice with no added sugar. Pomegranate juice contains a lot of naturally occurring sugar, so dilute two to four ounces of juice with an equal amount of water. Drink it with meals to slow the absorption of sugar into the bloodstream and help to maintain stable blood glucose levels. Use twice daily.

THE RIGHT REGIMEN FOR YOU

Arterial plaque buildup can be detected and its severity gauged using imaging tests, such as *computed tomography* (CT), *magnetic resonance imaging* (MRI) scan and/or ultrasound. Results help to determine the appropriate therapy for you. Tests may be repeated periodically to see if your regimen needs to be modified.

The four natural substances described in this article, used alone or in combination (following the dosage guidelines in the main article), can improve the health of your arteries. *Here's how to tell which ones are right for you...*

Note: If you take blood-thinning medication, talk to your doctor before using these substances.

- **If you do not have atherosclerosis, take one or more of these...**
  - Vitamin K.
  - Aged garlic extract (AGE).
  - Pomegranate juice.

- **For mild atherosclerosis, take all of these...**
  - Vitamin K.
  - AGE.
  - Pomegranate juice.

- **For moderate or severe atherosclerosis, take all of these...**
  - Tocotrienols.
  - Vitamin K.
  - AGE.
  - Pomegranate juice.
  - Statin medication—but only if you and your doctor are not satisfied with your level of improvement after 12 months of daily use of all four natural substances.

REPORT #3
Could This B Vitamin Boost Your Hearing?

American Academy of Otolaryngology—Head and Neck Surgery news release

Low levels of folic acid (folate) may be associated with age-related hearing loss, says a recent study.

BACKGROUND

Hearing loss affects more than 28 million Americans aged 60 to 74. Despite that high prevalence, little is known about the biological basis of age-related hearing loss, researchers say.

A study that followed 126 healthy Nigerian men and women over age 60 found that low serum levels of folic acid, a B vitamin, were significantly associated with hearing loss in high frequencies.

The finding appears in an issue of the journal *Otolaryngology—Head and Neck Surgery*.

"Based on our research, age-related hearing loss may be associated with poor micronutrient status. The role of folate in cellular metabolism, the nervous system, and vascular function are important for the auditory system," study author Akeem Olawale Lasisi said in a journal news release.

FURTHER RESEARCH NEEDED

The researchers called for further study into the role of vitamins in hearing, particularly in developing countries where malnutrition is common.

Folic acid is found in fruits; leafy green vegetables, such as romaine lettuce; dried beans; peas; nuts, and enriched cereals and breads. It is also available as a dietary supplement.

For more about hearing loss, visit the Web site of the US National Institute on Aging, *www.nia.nih.gov*. Type "hearing loss" into the search box.

REPORT #4
The New Anticancer Formula

Raymond Chang, MD, faculty member at Weill Cornell Medical College, New York City, and a pioneer in the use of complementary and alternative treatments in oncology. He is author of *Beyond the Magic Bullet—The Anti-Cancer Cocktail: A New Approach to Beating Cancer* (Square One).

Researchers are discovering that multiple treatments given simultaneously can be far more effective at fighting cancer than any single treatment. That's because a typical cancer involves an average of 63 genetic mutations, each of which works in different ways. A single treatment is unlikely to affect more than a few of these processes.

Better approach: Cancer "cocktails" that simultaneously attack abnormal cells in a multitude of ways.

Examples: A deadly form of blood cancer, multiple myeloma, now is routinely treated with drug combinations that have doubled survival rates. A French study, published in the *New England Journal of Medicine*, found that patients with pancreatic cancer who were given a combination of four drugs lived about 60% longer than those given standard chemotherapy.

For the most part, the conventional treatment strategy for cancer involves using one or two traditional treatments—surgery, radiation, chemotherapy or hormone therapy—one after the other. Only on occasion are different treatments used in combination simultaneously such as when radiation and chemotherapy are administered following a patient's surgery.

Many oncologists now believe that it's better to hit cancers all at once with a barrage of treatments—including, in some cases, unconventional treatments, such as vitamins, herbs, supplements and medications typically prescribed for other health problems.

Example: I might advise a cancer patient getting conventional treatments to include the arthritis drug *celecoxib* (Celebrex), which makes cancer cells more sensitive to radiation…the hormone melatonin (which decreases the growth of some cancers)…and vitamin D-3 (which may reduce cancer recurrence).

GETTING STARTED

Here's how to make this approach work for you…

• **Keep an open mind.** Ask your doctor if there are safe and effective treatments that he/she recommends that may be unconventional, including "off-label" drugs—medications that haven't been approved by the FDA specifically for your type of cancer. Doctors often know about new treatments that seem to work for a given cancer.

Important: Don't try any treatment without first checking with your doctor to make sure that it is safe for you. If it is, he/she can recommend the right dose and tell you when you should take it.

• **Start with conventional care.** I never advise patients to forgo appropriate standard cancer treatments such as chemotherapy and/or radiation. These approaches have been proven to improve survival. You can then supplement these approaches with off-label medications, herbs and/or supplements to help increase effectiveness.

• **Define your goals.** A cure isn't the only reason to use a medley of treatments. The right cocktail also can reduce treatment side effects and improve your quality of life.

Example: Patients with breast cancer may be given hormonal treatments that reduce tumor growth, but in premenopausal women, these treatments also induce early menopause—and the accompanying hot flashes, night sweats and "brain fog." To be more comfortable during the post-treatment period, you can take vitamin E to reduce hot flashes…ginkgo to improve memory…and herbs such as black cohosh to reduce vaginal dryness and night sweats.

INGREDIENTS TO CONSIDER

Ask your doctor what you can add to your current treatments to increase their effectiveness. Some of the most common medications in the US have been shown to help cancer patients, as have supplements. *Here, some unconventional treatments that can help…*

• **Vitamin D.** Studies have shown that vitamin D induces *apoptosis*, the death of cancer cells. This is important because one of the characteristics of cancer cells is the ability to avoid cell death. Using vitamin D along with chemotherapy, surgery and/or radiation could improve your outcome.

• **The ulcer medication *cimetidine*** (Tagamet) strengthens the immune system so that it can fight cancer cells. Studies have shown that patients who start taking cimetidine a few days before colon cancer surgery may be less likely to have a recurrence of the cancer.

• **Aspirin.** An analysis of data from the Harvard Nurses' Health Study found that breast cancer patients who took aspirin reduced the risk of the cancer spreading (metastasis) by nearly 50%.

• **Curcumin,** the active compound in the spice turmeric. Like aspirin, it's an anti-inflammatory that can reduce the invasion and spread of cancer cells. It also can inhibit *angiogenesis*, the development of blood vessels that nourish tumors.

• **Green tea.** This is one cancer-cocktail ingredient that everyone can "take." One cup of green tea has approximately 45 milligrams (mg) of *epigallocatechin 3-gallate* (EGCG), a compound that appears to reduce the growth of cancer cells. Dozens of studies have shown that green tea may be effective.

Example: A Mayo Clinic study found that the majority of leukemia patients who took EGCG showed clear improvement. Other studies have shown that it can reduce prostate-specific antigen (PSA), a substance that is elevated in patients with prostate cancer.

I recommend eight cups of green tea a day to fight cancer.

• **Red yeast rice.** This type of yeast, taken in supplement form, contains monacolin K, the same active compound that is used in lovastatin, one of the cholesterol-lowering statins. Red yeast rice is an anti-inflammatory that also affects immune response and cell signaling—actions that can help prevent and possibly treat some cancers.

Laboratory studies indicate that red yeast rice (as well as statins) might increase the effectiveness of radiation and chemotherapy.

As for statins, in studies involving nearly a half-million patients, the drugs have been shown to significantly reduce the incidence and recurrence of colon, breast, lung and prostate cancers.

GO SLOW

Mix the cocktail slowly. It's not good to start many treatments at the same time. You need to know if a particular ingredient is causing side effects.

Example: I might advise a patient to use Chinese herbs for a week. If he/she is doing well, I might add a second ingredient and then a third.

REPORT #5
Alternatives for Uncomfortable Sleep Apnea Treatments

David M. Rapoport, MD, associate professor of medicine and director of the sleep medicine program at New York University School of Medicine, New York City.

If you're one of the 18 million Americans who have been diagnosed with moderate-to-severe sleep apnea, chances are your doctor has suggested that you try a continuous positive airway pressure, or CPAP (pronounced "SEE-pap"), machine.

Problem: Many people complain that the CPAP face mask is too uncomfortable to wear and often causes problems such as mouth dryness.

Solution: There are now many ways to make CPAP treatment less uncomfortable—or, if necessary, you can use one of various alternative therapies that are effective when CPAP is not tolerated.

WHAT IS SLEEP APNEA?

Sleep apnea occurs when breathing temporarily stops multiple times during sleep. Symptoms may include snoring, gasping, choking and daytime drowsiness. At least 10% of adults over age 65 are believed to have the most common form, obstructive sleep apnea, though the majority of them don't know it. The condition affects men and women.

THE SLEEP APNEA CHALLENGE

Sleep apnea frequently goes undiagnosed. Even though snoring is a telltale symptom in some sufferers, not everyone who snores has sleep apnea—and not everyone with sleep apnea snores.

Red flag: If you have chronic snoring loud enough to wake your bed partner, you may have sleep apnea.

Don't ignore this condition: If you have moderate-to-severe sleep apnea (20 or more interruptions in breathing per night), be sure to seek medical treatment. Sleep apnea causes severe sleepiness and has been linked to impaired cognitive function (including memory loss), elevated blood pressure, increased stroke and heart attack risk and a higher mortality rate.

CPAP—IF YOU CAN TOLERATE IT

Use of a CPAP machine is widely considered the most effective treatment for moderate-to-severe sleep apnea. If you're overweight, weight loss also helps.

CPAP increases the pressure of the air being breathed, which helps keep the airway open. The CPAP machine—about the size of a dictionary—pumps air into a hose that is connected to a face mask (nasal or full-face covering the nose and mouth). *Modifications that make CPAP more user-friendly include…*

•**More comfortable mask designs** are available in a variety of designs from Respironics…ResMed…and Fisher & Paykel Healthcare, as well as from specialty manufacturers, such as Dreamweaver and CPAP Pro.

•**Humidifying feature to fight mouth dryness**—some CPAP machines are built with features to maximally humidify or to allow an external humidifier to be attached, while others come with an internal humidifier. Humidifying CPAP machines and attachments can be found at *www.directhomemedical.com*, 888-505-0212.

•**Bilevel positive airway pressure** (BiPAP and others) and C-Flex are modified versions of CPAP that reduce air pressure as the wearer exhales, which some patients find more comfortable. (CPAP provides constant and steady air pressure, whereas bilevel devices provide varying pressure.) Bilevel machines cost more than those used for CPAP, starting at about $1,700 versus about $800.

New: CPAP can be modified with a breathing sensor called SensAwake that detects when the user's breathing pattern becomes irregular (indicating partial wakefulness) and drops the pressure.* The CPAP resumes full pressure only when regular breathing indicates the patient is asleep. CPAP machines with built-in SensAwake technology are manufactured by Fisher & Paykel Healthcare and are available at *www.cpap.com* (800-356-5221).

CPAP ALTERNATIVES

If you still find CPAP too uncomfortable to use, consider…

•**Oral appliances.** These hinged mouthpieces, which are worn during sleep, pull the lower jaw (and base of the tongue) forward to keep the upper airway open. Oral appliances are typically custom-made by a dentist. The initial cost of an oral appliance (usually about $1,000) is similar to that of CPAP, but patients usually need a half dozen follow-up dentist visits to adjust the appliance.

•**Nasal devices.** Provent (Ventus Medical) is a disposable device that's attached to the nostrils at night, then thrown away in the morning. The opening of the device narrows during exhalation, which increases pressure in the airway. It is believed that this makes the airway less prone to collapse. Provent, which must be prescribed by a doctor, was recently approved by the FDA.

The good news: It costs just $2 a day ($730 a year) and can easily be tried for a week.

•**Sleep position products.** Sleep apnea worsens when the sufferer is lying on his/her back. That's because gravity makes it more likely that throat muscles will collapse and block the person's airway.

Products that help people stay off their backs during sleep include an "antisnore" T-shirt (with pockets sewn on the back to hold inflatable or Styrofoam "bumpers"). It is available from Rematee, 877-753-6844, *www.antisnoreshirt.com*. Or sew a pocket on the back of a T-shirt and place a tennis ball inside.

Several pillows that are designed to promote side sleeping also are available.

Examples: Sona Pillow, $79.99...and Splintek Sleep Right Side Sleeping Pillow, $65.00* both available at *www.amazon.com*

SURGERY: A LAST RESORT

If noninvasive approaches don't relieve sleep apnea symptoms, there are surgical options. These include a procedure that removes tissue from the throat and mouth (with a success rate of up to 40%) and another that remolds the lower and upper jaw to increase airway space (with a success rate of up to 90%).

Exciting new approach: An experimental implant, which is about the size of a matchbox and known as a hypoglossal nerve stimulator, is implanted under the collarbone to electrically stimulate the throat's nerves so that the tissues won't collapse and block the airway.

The implant has shown promising results in early trials but is not yet available.

One catch: The battery needs replacing every three to five years, requiring another small operation.

REPORT #6
The Accidental Cure for High Blood Pressure

Nicholas D. Schiff, MD, director, Laboratory of Cognitive Neuromodulation, New York-Presbyterian Hospital/Weill Cornell Medical Center, New York City.

Marc Penn, MD, cardiologist, former director, Bakken Heart-Brain Institute, Cleveland Clinic, Cleveland, Ohio.

Neurology

Doctors administering deep brain stimulation to control a patient's severe pain report that they discovered the treatment consistently lowered the man's hard-to-control high blood pressure.

The finding introduces the possibility that deep brain stimulation—a surgical implant that delivers electrical pulses to the brain—might one day become a treatment for drug-resistant hypertension or lead to clues about the brain's role in regulating blood pressure.

The study was reported in the journal *Neurology*.

TOUGH-TO-CONTROL BLOOD PRESSURE

About 10% of high blood pressure cases either can't be controlled with drugs or patients cannot tolerate them, study author Dr. Nikunj K. Patel, a neurosurgeon at Frenchay Hospital in Bristol, England, said in a journal news release.

According to the US Centers for Disease Control and Prevention, high blood pressure affects 30% of American adults. The condition raises the risk of heart attack and stroke.

"It's a really interesting paper," said Nicholas D. Schiff, MD, director of the Laboratory of Cognitive Neuromodulation at New York-Presbyterian Hospital/Weill Cornell Medical Center. "I thought it was compelling, though single cases are always questionable" to generalize from.

THE DISCOVERY

In the case study, a 55-year-old man was implanted with a deep brain stimulator to treat severe pain stemming from a stroke. Although the patient was taking four drugs to control his high blood pressure, which was diagnosed at the time of his stroke, his blood pressure had remained high.

The man's blood pressure gradually decreased enough for him to stop taking all blood pressure medications, though the deep brain stimulation failed to control his pain long-term. When researchers tested turning off the stimulator after two years, the patient's blood pressure rose significantly.

The study adds to other recent research focused on neuromodulation, which harnesses the power of electrical impulses in the body for therapeutic benefit. Tactics being tested include renal nerve ablation, a procedure that emits low-power radiofrequency along the nerves next to the kidneys, interrupting signals that trigger high blood pressure.

*Prices are subject to change.

MORE EXPERT REACTION

"In the general sense, neuromodulation for blood pressure is really going to be a revolutionary treatment for chronic [high] blood pressure," said cardiologist Marc Penn, MD, former director of the Cleveland Clinic's Bakken Heart-Brain Institute.

"I think it's really interesting physiology," added Dr. Penn, noting that the results would need to be repeated multiple times before a therapy based on it could be developed.

Dr. Schiff, however, was hesitant to predict that deep brain stimulation might become a common treatment for hard-to-control high blood pressure.

"This is a case report, and not a treatment for anything," he said, adding, "There are risks to this procedure and one has to really look at the tradeoffs."

For more information about deep brain stimulation, visit the Web site of the American Association of Neurological Surgeons, *www.aans.org*, and type "deep brain stimulation" into the search box.

REPORT #7
Pop a Purple Potato to Lower Blood Pressure

In a recent study, 18 overweight people with high blood pressure ate about seven golf ball–sized purple potatoes twice daily for a month. The potatoes with skins were cooked in a microwave.

Result: The study participants' diastolic (bottom number) blood pressure readings dropped 4%, on average, and their systolic (top number) readings were 3.5% lower. None of the participants gained weight. Purple potatoes are available at specialty-food stores and some supermarkets.

Joe Vinson, PhD, professor of chemistry, The University of Scranton, Pennsylvania.

REPORT #8
More Than 80% of Blood Pressure Readings Are Wrong

Steven Burgess, MD, chief resident in family medicine at Texas Tech University Health Sciences Center, School of Medicine, Amarillo.

Here's a disturbing bit of news. A recent study reports that 81% of blood pressure measurements taken by doctors and nurses are done improperly, resulting in numerous misdiagnoses. This means that many people are taking medications that they really don't need!

The American Heart Association has published guidelines recommending a particular methodology to follow when taking blood pressure measurements in a clinical setting, such as a doctor's office. In an earlier study, researchers evaluated pressure-taking techniques of 172 doctors and nurses and reported that none were following guidelines set by the American Heart Association—this inspired Steven Burgess, MD, chief resident in family medicine at Texas Tech University Health Sciences Center, School of Medicine in Amarillo, to undertake a study to evaluate how these potentially erroneous measurements impact patient care.

What he learned is disconcerting. He said that the mistakes made when taking blood pressure readings were significant enough to change treatment recommendations for more than half the patients in the study! "My study showed that if someone initially has elevated blood pressure and we redo the reading in accordance with the guidelines, over 50% of the time the new 'correct' pressure puts the patient into a different category, which would cause treatment to be different," he said, noting that the pressure is virtually always lower when taken "correctly."

MISTAKES ARE MADE

The most common blood pressure measurement mistake being made by health-care practitioners is to take a blood pressure reading immediately after a patient sits down. The guidelines say that patients should rest quietly for five minutes first. Why? Because physical activity raises blood pressure, often by 10 mmHg or more.

In his 18-month study of 56 patients, Dr. Burgess found that when blood pressure is measured properly, the average patient's systolic (top number) reading is 15.7 mmHg lower than when the guidelines aren't being followed. For more than half (56.4%) of the patients, using the correct technique—compared with doing it the wrong way—meant that patients were fine without medication or changes to their current therapy.

MEASURE BY MEASURE

Here are the American Heart Association's guidelines regarding the proper technique for measuring blood pressure…

- **Patients should not exercise, drink caffeine or smoke for 30 minutes** prior to measurement and should sit quietly for five minutes immediately before.

- **While the measurement is being taken, the patient should be comfortably seated with his/her back supported** (not perched on a stool or a table) and with feet flat on the floor. The patient's bare arm (the sleeve can be rolled up or, if it is too constricting, the shirt can be removed) should be supported at the level of his heart. In other words, the patient should lean his arm on an armrest or table or the doctor or nurse taking the reading should hold the patient's arm, not let it hang at the patient's side.

- **The cuff must fit properly according to specific guidelines.** For most people, a standard cuff will satisfy these guidelines, but large or obese patients or those who are unusually small require special-sized equipment.

For professional equipment (what's used by a health-care professional), the cuff should be placed one inch above the elbow. For digital monitors designed to be used at home, the cuff should be centered over the inside of the elbow.

- **No talking—by either the patient or the practitioner.** Speaking not only raises blood pressure, it also interferes with the practitioner's ability to focus on your pulse while taking a reading.

- **At an initial visit, two readings should be taken and the results should be averaged.** If the readings differ by more than 5 mmHg, a third reading should be taken and averaged with the other two. (*Note*: At subsequent visits, a single reading may be sufficient.)

HOMEWORK

Lots of people now monitor their blood pressure at home—so it's important that everyone recognizes that these readings must be done in the proper way. Be sure you are using the right type of equipment and following instructions. Also check to see whether your equipment gives you readings that match those taken in your doctor's office.

REPORT #9

FDA Approves Drug That Shows Promise for Certain Breast Cancers

Kimberly Blackwell, MD, professor of medicine and an assistant professor of radiation oncology at Duke Cancer Institute in Durham, North Carolina.

Daniel F. Hayes, MD, clinical director, Breast Oncology Program, University of Michigan Comprehensive Cancer Center, Ann Arbor.

American Society of Clinical Oncology, news release

An experimental drug designed to treat patients with a specific kind of breast cancer known as HER2-positive appeared to boost survival compared with a standard treatment, a recent study shows.

The drug, known as *trastuzumab emtansine* (T-DM1), was recently approved for marketing by the US Food and Drug Administration (February 2013).

Patients with HER2-positive breast cancer have a protein called *human epidermal growth factor receptor 2* that promotes cancer cell growth.

The drug T-DM1 is a dual drug made up of the antibody *trastuzumab* (Herceptin) and the cytotoxic drug *emtansine* (DM1).

STUDY DETAILS

In the study, nearly 1,000 patients received either T-DM1 or a regimen of *capecitabine* (Xeloda) and *lapatinib* (Tykerb), a combination referred to as XL. They took the assigned treatment until the disease got worse or side effects became unmanageable.

After two years, 65.4% of those who took T-DM1 were alive, compared with 47.5% of those who took the other treatment.

The median progression-free survival time was 9.6 months for those who got T-DM1, compared with 6.4 months for the others.

The T-DM1 regimen was generally well tolerated by study participants, the researchers said. Those who got the standard treatment were more likely to experience diarrhea, stomach upset and redness, swelling and pain in their palms and the soles of their feet.

MORE EFFECTIVE, LESS TOXIC

Daniel Hayes, MD, clinical director of the breast oncology program at the University of Michigan Comprehensive Cancer Center in Ann Arbor, said the study suggests that T-DM1 will provide us with yet another effective and meaningful agent to use in women with HER2-positive breast cancer.

"The drug worked. It was significantly better than a very effective approved therapy for HER2-overexpressing metastatic breast cancer," said study author Kimberly Blackwell, MD, a professor of medicine and an assistant professor of radiation oncology at Duke Cancer Institute in Durham, North Carolina.

"Also, as a clinician who takes care of a lot of breast cancer patients, I'm pleased that this drug has very little dose-limiting toxicity," she added. "Patients don't lose their hair from this drug. For patients facing metastatic breast cancer, this is a breakthrough."

REPORT #10
Pain Killer Lowers Breast Cancer Recurrence

The painkiller a woman takes after a mastectomy may influence the odds of breast cancer recurrence, a recent study suggests.

STUDY DETAILS

Researchers at the Catholic University of Louvain in Belgium looked for links between painkiller use and breast cancer recurrence in 327 women from one to four years after they underwent a mastectomy.

Women who received a powerful prescription nonsteroidal anti-inflammatory drug (NSAID) called *ketorolac* (sold as Toradol and Acular) which is related to aspirin and ibuprofen, were less likely to develop a recurrence of breast cancer. Their rate was 6% compared with 17% for those who received other drugs for pain.

The link between the painkiller and lower rate of recurrence remained even after the researchers adjusted for factors such as patient age and stage of cancer.

The study was published in the journal *Anesthesia & Analgesia*.

For more about breast cancer, visit the Web site of the National Cancer Institute, *www.cancer.gov/cancertopics/pdq/treatment/breast/patient*.

International Anesthesia Research Society, press release

REPORT #11
Eat Dark Meat for a Healthier Heart

Dark meat may lower coronary heart disease (CHD) risk.

Background: Taurine is a nutrient found in the dark meat of chicken and turkey as well as in some fish and shellfish.

Recent study: Researchers took blood samples to measure levels of taurine in 223 women (average age 59) with CHD.

Finding: Women with high cholesterol and high levels of taurine were 60% less likely to develop CHD over a 20-year period than similar women with low taurine levels.

Yu Chen, PhD, MPH, associate professor of epidemiology, New York University School of Medicine, New York City.

REPORT #12
The Instant Migraine Eraser

Marvin Mansky, DDS, New York City.
Stephen Silberstein, MD, professor of neurology, Jefferson Medical College, and director, Jefferson Headache Center, Thomas Jefferson University, Philadelphia.

Can a mouth device prevent your head from throbbing? Maybe. The US Food and Drug Administration (FDA) has approved the *nociceptive trigeminal inhibition-tension suppression system* (NTI-tss) for the prevention of migraine and tension-type headache pain.

Marvin Mansky, DDS, a Manhattan dentist, admits he didn't think much of the idea at first. But now, after he's used it to treat 350 patients (and wears one himself occasionally), he's a believer.

"It reduces the frequency and intensity of migraines dramatically," Dr. Mansky says. "For some, it stops the migraines completely."

THE DEVICE

Made of clear plastic, the inch-wide NTI device fits over two front teeth—usually, but not always, the top teeth.

It prevents the teeth from clenching—which the developer of the device, also a dentist, claims is the cause of many headaches.

According to the proponents of the NTI device, prolonged, intense clenching stresses the temporal muscles that open and close the jaw, often triggering migraine as well as tension headaches.

The first person Dr. Mansky fitted with one was a woman who had severe head pain. Her pain was reduced immediately, he said. And within two weeks, all pain was gone.

For that relief, many people seem willing to pay roughly $750 for the tiny tooth protector. Dr. Mansky and other dentists around the country can mold and custom-fit the device in about an hour. Most people wear it only while sleeping, although some wear a slightly less obtrusive device during the day as well.

ANOTHER OPINION

However, Stephen Silberstein, MD, a professor of neurology at Thomas Jefferson University in Philadelphia, disputes the connection between clenching and headaches.

"There's scientific evidence to show that only rarely does clenching ever produce headaches," Dr. Silberstein says.

Although he is unfamiliar with this particular device, Dr. Silberstein says it's "logical" that if it stops people from grinding their teeth, it would relieve any pain that stems from teeth grinding.

Responding to the criticism, the inventor of the device—California dentist James P. Boyd, DDS—cites an Irish study that showed the jaw-clenching muscles in people who experience migraines were nearly 70% larger, as well as stronger, than the same muscles in people who did not have migraines. Dr. Boyd believes that points to a clear link between clenching and migraine headaches.

For more about headaches, check the Web site of the American Headache Society at *www.achenet.org*.

REPORT #13
Injection Helps Cancer Patients Live Pain Free

Giovanni Carlo Anselmetti, MD, Institute for Cancer Research and Treatment, Turin, Italy.

Mark Montgomery, MD, associate professor, radiology, Texas A&M Health Science Center College of Medicine, Temple, Texas, and director, interventional radiology, and vice chair, education in radiology, Scott & White Healthcare, Temple, Texas.

Susan Bukata, MD, associate professor, orthopaedics, University of Rochester Medical Center, New York.

Society for Interventional Radiology annual meeting, San Diego.

Injecting "bone cement" into areas of weakened bone in patients whose cancer has spread to their bones can literally allow these individuals to rise from their deathbeds and live the remainder of their lives relatively pain free.

Italian researchers, who presented the findings at the Society of Interventional Radiology annual meeting in San Diego, called it the "Lazarus Effect," referring to when Jesus miraculously raised Lazarus from the dead.

"The majority of treated patients experienced significant or complete and long-lasting pain relief after osteoplasty with immediate improvement of clinical conditions and quality of life," said study author Giovanni Carlo Anselmetti, MD, of the Institute for Cancer Research and Treatment in Turin.

Indeed, a 79-year-old nun who was confined to her bed because of thyroid cancer that had spread to her pelvis stood and walked just two hours after the minimally invasive procedure.

BACKGROUND

Orthopedists who do osteoplasty generally partner with an interventional radiologist who first performs radiofrequency ablation (extreme heat) or cryoablation (freezing) to kill nerve cells near the tumor.

Osteoplasty involves injecting bone cement (they used *polymethyl-methacrylate*, or PMMA, in the study) into bony areas weakened by cancer with the help of a computed tomography (CT) scan or other image guidance.

"The procedure is analogous to vertebroplasty, which has been around for a few years, where you put little needles into the spine and inject a cement mixture," said Mark Montgomery, MD, an associate professor of radiology at Texas A&M Health Science Center College of Medicine and director of interventional radiology and vice chair of education in radiology at Scott & White Healthcare. "It uses the same kind of cement as for total hip replacement. This is the same thing, except they're just taking it into other areas," he added.

THE STUDY

The recent study involved 81 patients, ages 36 to 94 and mostly female, who underwent osteoplasty at least once. Seventy-four of the participants had cancer, while a handful had "benign" diseases, such as rheumatoid arthritis.

The overall patient population was larger than those seen in other studies, said Susan Bukata, MD, an orthopedic oncologist at the University of Rochester Medical Center.

Pelvic, femur, sacrum, ribs, knee and other bones were treated.

THE RESULTS

The mean pain score dropped significantly within 24 hours of the procedure. Sixty-four of the patients (79%) were able to discontinue use of narcotics and 43 (53%) also stopped using any other pain medications. Only five of the patients showed no improvement in pain. There were no deaths or major complications.

PAIN CONTROL OPTION

"It is palliative. It's not going to be a curative procedure, but we've seen dramatic improvements in pain control," said Dr. Montgomery. "There's a lack of an awareness of some of the options for patients that have painful bone metastases," he added. "It's physician education as much as it is patient education."

REPORT #14
Keep Your Hair During Chemo

Breast cancer patients are more likely to keep their hair when scalp-cooling caps are worn during chemo sessions, reports Hope Rugo, MD. The Penguin Cold Cap contains a frozen gel that cools the scalp, reducing blood flow to the area and minimizing chemo's effect on the scalp. The cap requires changing every 20 minutes (more convenient models are under development).

Information: *www.penguincoldcaps.com.*

Hope Rugo, MD, codirector of the breast oncology clinical trials program and clinical professor of medicine, Helen Diller Family Comprehensive Cancer Center, University of California, San Francisco.

REPORT #15
Reduce Your Breast Cancer Risk by 23%

Lila Nachtigall, MD, professor, obstetrics and gynecology, NYU Langone Medical Center, New York City.

Garnet Anderson, PhD, principal investigator, Women's Health Initiative Clinical Coordinating Center, Fred Hutchinson Cancer Research Center, Seattle.

Stephanie Bernik, MD, chief, surgical oncology, Lenox Hill Hospital, New York City.

The Lancet Oncology, online

Some women who take estrogen-only hormone replacement therapy to stave off hot flashes, night sweats and other symptoms of menopause may be at lower risk for developing breast cancer down the road, a recent study says.

BACKGROUND

Hormone replacement therapy (HRT) fell from grace rather dramatically after a large government-run trial, the US Women's Health Initiative, was stopped early in 2002 because HRT was shown to increase the risk of strokes and breast and ovarian cancer. Since that time, however, some subtleties have emerged as researchers parsed the evidence further. For example, short-term use of HRT is now deemed fairly safe for some women who have severe menopausal symptoms.

RECENT FINDINGS

The study shows that longer-term use of estrogen-only therapy may actually lower a woman's odds of developing breast cancer. Estrogen-only therapy is reserved for women who have had a hysterectomy; women with an intact uterus who use HRT must take the hormone progestin with estrogen to prevent uterine cancer.

"Women who have had a hysterectomy may be reassured that taking estrogen by itself, short term, to relieve menopausal symptoms will not increase their risk of breast cancer," said study author Garnet Anderson, PhD, of the Women's Health Initiative Clinical Coordinating Center at the Fred Hutchinson Cancer Research Center in Seattle. Women should not take estrogen to prevent breast cancer, she stressed.

The findings were published in an online edition of *The Lancet Oncology.*

The North American Menopause Society recently released a position statement that backs up these findings. The group said starting combination hormone therapy (both estrogen and progestin) around the time of menopause to treat symptoms and stave off the brittle-bone disease osteoporosis is safe for some women for three to five years. Estrogen alone can be used for longer than the combination HRT, according to the society.

STUDY DETAILS

The study, which was partially funded by drug manufacturer Wyeth (which is now a part of Pfizer Inc.), included more than 7,500 women from the Women's Health Initiative who took estrogen for about six years. Roughly five years after stopping treatment, the women were 23% less likely to develop breast cancer when compared with their counterparts who never used HRT.

Women in the estrogen group who did develop breast cancer were 63% less likely to die from the disease, compared with women who never took it. The lower risk of breast cancer was seen only among women without risk factors for breast cancer, such as a history of benign breast disease or a strong family history of breast cancer, the study showed.

IMPLICATIONS

"The story is pretty clear about estrogen plus progestin—no matter the age of the women, estrogen plus progestin increases [the risk of] breast cancer, heart disease, stroke and blood clots," Dr. Anderson said. "These risks outweigh the benefits for all age groups."

Why estrogen alone may lower breast cancer risk while adding progestin seems to increase the risk is the million-dollar question.

"There are hypotheses about the role of estrogen in breasts after a woman has gone through menopause," Dr. Anderson said. For example, "her breast tissue, including any precancerous cells, may go through changes as a result of menopause that make them susceptible to estrogen in a way that discourages cell growth."

Estrogen-only therapy is not without risks, however. For estrogen alone, the Women's Health Initiative data showed no overall effect of estrogen on heart disease, but an increased risk of strokes and blood clots.

RECOMMENDATIONS

Women are understandably confused about whether they should take hormones to treat their menopausal symptoms, and for how long they can safely use the therapy.

"The best use of estrogen-alone is in women with a hysterectomy who need relief of hot flashes and night sweats and related menopausal symptoms," Dr. Anderson said. These benefits need to be weighed against a woman's risk of stroke or developing blood clots.

Lila Nachtigall, MD, a professor of obstetrics and gynecology at NYU Langone Medical Center in New York City, agreed that, when used on its own, estrogen can still be safe and effective in treating the symptoms of menopause in women who do not have a uterus.

"It looks very definite that the bad guy is progestin, not estrogen," Dr. Nachtigall said. Her advice is to use the lowest effective dose for the shortest amount of time. If more women took estrogen, she said, there would be a dent made in the epidemic of osteoporosis. "Millions of women who never went on estrogen, even for a few years, are really losing bone," she said.

IMPORTANT

That said, estrogen does increase the risk for blood clots. "Women with blood-clotting disorders should not take it," Dr. Nachtigall said.

Commenting on the study, Stephanie Bernik, MD, chief of surgical oncology at Lenox Hill Hospital in New York City, said, "If you are looking to reduce menopausal symptoms and don't have an intact uterus, [estrogen] is an option." But estrogen-only therapy should not be prescribed indiscriminately, she added.

"This applies only to women who have severe menopausal symptoms. We are not saying that we should give women estrogen to reduce the risk of breast cancer," Dr. Bernik added.

Learn more about the benefits and risks of hormone therapy at the North American Menopause Society's Web site, *www.menopause.org* (search "hormone therapy risks").

REPORT #16
Fish Oil Works as Well as Drugs to Treat Depression

Results of the largest-ever trial of omega-3 supplements for depression, the Omega-3D Trial, found that fish oil supplements (1,050 milligrams [mg] daily of *eicosapentaenoic acid*, or EPA) improved depression symptoms as much as is reported by those taking prescription drugs—particularly those with major depression who did not also have an anxiety disorder. Speak to a physician about switching from a prescription medication to fish oil that has at least 1,050 mg of EPA, the component that helps depression. The amount of *docosahexaenoic acid* (DHA) doesn't affect depression.

Mark A. Stengler, NMD, naturopathic medical doctor and leading authority on the practice of alternative and integrated medicine. Dr. Stengler is author of the *Health Revelations* newsletter, author of *The Natural Physician's Healing Therapies* (Bottom Line Books), founder and medical director of the Stengler Center for Integrative Medicine in Encinitas, California, and adjunct associate clinical professor at the National College of Natural Medicine in Portland, Oregon. *http://markstengler.com*

REPORT #17
Pumpkin Seeds Boost Mood

Like chocolate, pumpkin seeds are a good source of the amino acid *tryptophan*, which improves mood—but pumpkin seeds don't have the sugar that chocolate does, and one ounce of pumpkin seeds contains about half the daily requirement of magnesium, which strengthens bones. Sprinkle toasted seeds on soups and salads, or put raw, unsalted seeds on the tops of muffins before baking.

Melina Jampolis, MD, physician nutrition specialist, San Francisco, and author of *The Busy Person's Guide to Permanent Weight Loss* (Thomas Nelson). Her Web site is www.drmelina.com.

REPORT #18
Fruit Conquers Jet Lag

Tart cherries—also known as sour cherries—have high levels of melatonin, which helps regulate your circadian rhythm and induce sleepiness.

Best: Have one-half cup of dried tart cherries (such as Montmorency) or two tablespoons of any cherry juice concentrate one hour before you wish to sleep on the plane and an hour before bedtime for the three days after you land.

Russel Reiter, PhD, professor of neuroendocrinology, University of Texas Health Science Center, San Antonio.

REPORT #19
Vitamin D Eases Breast Cancer Drug Pain

Antonella Luisa Rastelli, MD, assistant professor of medicine in the section of medical oncology at Washington University School of Medicine in St. Louis, and leader of a study of 60 breast cancer patients.

Drugs called *aromatase inhibitors,* which are used to treat breast cancer, can make muscles and joints so painful and stiff that some women taking the medications say that they feel like they're 100 years old…many users experience bone loss, too. Yet because the medication is effective at halting breast cancer cell growth, shrinking tumors and reducing recurrence risk when taken for several years or more, discontinuing its use prematurely often is inadvisable.

Recent study: Recognizing that many breast cancer patients have low blood levels of vitamin D, Antonella Luisa Rastelli, MD, an assistant professor of medicine in the section of medical oncology at Washington University School of Medicine in St. Louis and her team of researchers tested a simple potential solution to the problem of drug side effects—vitamin D supplements.

STUDY DETAILS

Participants included 60 early-stage breast cancer patients with low vitamin D levels who had painful side effects from the aromatase inhibitor *anastrozole* (Arimidex). All received a standard daily dose of 400 international units (IU) of vitamin D-3 (the type typically found in supplements) and 1,000 mg of calcium. Half of the participants also received 50,000 IU of vitamin D-2 (a form that leaves the body more quickly than D-3) weekly for eight or 16 weeks, then monthly to the end of the six-month study period. The other half, serving as the control group, got a placebo weekly or monthly.

Results: After two months of weekly supplementation, the high-dose vitamin D groups reported significantly less musculoskeletal pain than the control group (though pain relief did not continue when participants switched to the monthly regimen).

Also: After six months, the high-dose vitamin D users showed no reduction in bone density, whereas the control group did have some bone loss.

Excessive vitamin D can have side effects of its own, including high levels of calcium in the urine that may increase the risk for kidney stones. Risks are thought to be lower with vitamin D-2 than with D-3—but even so, Dr. Rastelli cautioned that all patients taking high-dose vitamin D supplements must be monitored closely, as the study participants were.

REPORT #20
Drinks That Melt Your Teeth

Bennett T. Amaechi, PhD, assistant professor, department of community dentistry at University of Texas Health Science Center, San Antonio.

Just when you think there can't possibly be any additional bad news about the ramifications of America's eating habits, here comes more. A recent study examined the teeth of 900 children between the ages of 10 and 14 in three different areas of the country.

The finding: 30% of the kids had dental erosion in which the enamel on the teeth begins to erode, leaving teeth thinner and less protected. Ironically, this erosion makes teeth smoother and shinier at first, so it is highly unlikely that people will notice the early stage of this destruction.

The study was done at the University of Texas Health Science Center at San Antonio in association with the University of California at San Francisco and Indiana University in Indianapolis. According to Bennett T. Amaechi, PhD, assistant professor, department of community dentistry, the erosion results from repeated exposure to certain drinks including soft drinks, fruit and sports drinks, some sweetened herbal tea drinks, beer salts (lime-flavored salts added to beer) and fruit-flavored candies, called Lucas candies, imported from Mexico. Even such "healthy" foods as citrus fruits and drinks like seltzer will erode enamel. All of these are acidic—and excessive acid eats the enamel off teeth.

WHAT IT TAKES TO REPAIR THE DAMAGE

The good news: Cutting back on the offending beverages stops the erosion, and over time saliva actually begins to remineralize the tooth surface…though never completely. If you don't stop, the erosion progresses and eventually causes great sensitivity and pain. Teeth may begin to lose their shape. This is yet another reason it is so important to have regular dental exam—the dentist can identify the problem in time for patients to put an end to their bad habits.

Dr. Amaechi advises limiting how often you have citric-based drinks. The worst possible habit is drinking sodas all day long. Instead, limit them to mealtimes or one during an afternoon or morning break. Best case scenario is to give up sugary fruit drinks or sports beverages completely. If you're not planning to give up a beverage that may be causing the erosion, consider sipping it through a straw to lessen contact with teeth.

Expert warning: Dr. Amaechi cautions people with erosion to avoid brushing immediately after eating or drinking the acidic product.

Helpful: Rinsing with a mouthwash that contains fluoride. Fluoride, too, is controversial, but according to Dr. Amaechi, the amount in mouthwash isn't enough to be a problem and it's helpful in remineralizing the damaged tooth surface.

REPORT #21
What's Killing Older Americans?

Robert J.F. Laheij, PhD, epidemiologist, Radboud University Nijmegen Medical Centre, the Netherlands.
George Pankey, MD, head, infectious disease research, Ochsner Clinic Foundation, New Orleans.
The Journal of the American Medical Association

Taking heartburn drugs for prolonged periods increases the risk of developing pneumonia, according to a Dutch study. According to study author Robert J.F. Laheij, PhD, an epidemiologist in the Netherlands, these drugs work by reducing the production of stomach acid. Less stomach acid lets more of the bacteria survive.

"There can be some kind of aspiration of bacteria into the airway," he explains. And while his study looked specifically at pneumonia, several previous studies have indicated an increase in other respiratory infections, such as influenza and bronchitis, from long-term use of heartburn drugs.

THE STUDY

In his study of more than 364,000 people in the Netherlands national health insurance program, Dr. Laheij found that compared with similar people who were not taking heartburn drugs, the risk of pneumonia was nearly double among those taking *proton pump inhibitors* for prolonged periods. The risk was almost 66% higher for people regularly taking histamine antagonists, another type of drug used to fight heartburn.

Proton pump inhibitors—Nexium, Prevacid, Prilosec, etc.—suppress approximately 90% of stomach acid production.

Histamine inhibitors work differently, blocking the histamine that stimulates acid production. They include *cimetidine* (Tagamet), *famotidine* (Pepcid), *nizatidine* (Axid) and *ranitidine* (Zantac).

INDISCRIMINATELY USED

Because some prescription heartburn medications are available in lower-priced generic forms, and others are sold over-the-counter, they are taken by millions. These drugs account for more than $20 billion in annual sales.

The easy availability of these heartburn medications is a big part of the problem, says Dr. Laheij. Two or three weeks of treatment is enough, but many people continue to take the medicine for much longer.

"My advice would be to use them as long as necessary and then stop them," he says.

"I don't think these drugs should be used indiscriminately, and I think they are," says George Pankey, MD, head of infectious disease research at the Ochsner Clinic Foundation in New Orleans.

"Your doctor needs to know what you are taking," he adds. "In this country, perhaps more than [in Europe], physicians do not know everything that a patient is taking, especially over-the-counter (OTC) medications. If you are taking a lot of OTC medications or supplements, tell your doctor."

REPORT #22
Test Predicts Lung Cancer Survival

Two recent studies involving a total of 1,439 early-stage lung cancer patients found that a new test, known as a *molecular assay*, correctly predicts whether a patient's odds of death within five years of lung cancer surgery are low, intermediate or high by measuring the activity of 14 genes in cancerous tissue.

Benefit: Knowing a patient's prognosis helps doctors determine whether standard postoperative treatments, such as chemotherapy, should be considered.

David Jablons, MD, professor of thoracic oncology, University of California, San Francisco.

REPORT #23
The Covered-Up Cause Of IBS

Nancy Kraft, RD, clinical dietitian, University of Iowa, Iowa City.

Theodore M. Bayless, MD, professor of medicine, Johns Hopkins University, Baltimore.

American College of Gastroenterology annual meeting, Baltimore.

Cutting back on sugar and fat makes sense for people trying to control their weight, but there may be another health benefit. Two studies suggest that fat and fructose, the sugar in fruits and honey (and also a component of high fructose corn syrup, or HFCS, that is used to sweeten many soft drinks and packaged foods), also can contribute to gastrointestinal discomfort.

Irritable bowel syndrome (IBS) is a common disorder of the intestines that leads to pain, gassiness, bloating and changes in bowel habits, according to the American Gastroenterological Association. The disorder can lead to constipation in some and diarrhea in others. Some people experience both.

In the first report, Nancy Kraft, a clinical dietitian from the University of Iowa, and her colleagues say some patients who have IBS are fructose-intolerant, and restricting that type of sugar can improve their symptoms.

Kraft says fructose intolerance often is an overlooked component of IBS.

Her colleague Dr. Young Choi says that, "A fructose-restricted diet significantly improved symptoms in some IBS patients. Fructose intolerance is yet another piece of the IBS puzzle."

THE STUDY

In the study, the 14 patients with IBS who followed a fructose-free diet for one year experienced a significant reduction in abdominal pain, bloating and diarrhea.

However, IBS symptoms remained the same for the 12 patients who did not stick with the diet, the researchers report.

Kraft believes these results are encouraging, because "people who limit their intake of fructose see their symptoms improve or disappear," but that further study is needed.

SECOND STUDY

Researchers from the Mayo Clinic in Rochester, Minnesota, led by Yuri Saito, MD, collected data on the diets of 221 adults, aged 20 to 50 years. Of these patients, 102 had gastrointestinal disorders and 119 were healthy.

The research team found that patients with IBS or dyspepsia (indigestion) reported eating more monounsaturated fats compared with healthy patients. These patients also ate fewer carbohydrates than their healthy counterparts.

The Mayo investigators concluded that "future studies are needed to determine whether fat intake causes gastrointestinal symptoms."

Theodore M. Bayless, MD, a professor of medicine at Johns Hopkins University, is not surprised that fat and fructose are linked with IBS and dyspepsia.

He notes that both fat and fructose are hard to digest and can aggravate both conditions. But Dr. Bayless does not believe that restricting fructose cures IBS...it may only relieve symptoms.

He advises patients to avoid fatty foods and foods that contain high levels of fructose, such as grapes, dates, honey and apple and pear juice. He also advises patients to check food labels for HFCS to limit intake of the sweetener and to increase fiber intake.

REPORT #24
Best Ways to Avoid Painful Diverticulitis

Jamison Starbuck, ND, naturopathic physician in family practice and a guest lecturer at the University of Montana, both in Missoula. She is past president of the American Association of Naturopathic Physicians and a contributing editor to *The Alternative Advisor: The Complete Guide to Natural Therapies* and *Alternative Treatments* (Time Life).

If you're over age 60, your chances are fifty-fifty that you have diverticulosis, a condition marked by numerous small pouches (diverticula) in the wall of the colon.

Virtually everyone over age 80 is affected by the disease, and even 10% of people age 41 to 60 have it.

The good news is that the vast majority of people with diverticulosis are symptom-free. The condition becomes a problem only when one or more of these pouches get inflamed, becoming diverticulitis—due, for example, to weakening of the gastrointestinal wall and/or poor diet. With diverticulitis, you are likely to experience a sudden onset of pain and tenderness in the lower left abdomen. Diarrhea or constipation and a fever can also occur, as well as rectal bleeding. Fortunately, diet and lifestyle can significantly reduce the likelihood of diverticulosis turning into diverticulitis. *My advice...*

• **Eat the right foods.** We now know that the old notion that diverticulitis is caused by small, fibrous foods is simply not true. Many doctors had believed that certain foods, such as poppy seeds, lodged in the diverticula and became inflamed. However, an 18-year study published in the *Journal of the American Medical Association* conclusively showed that eating foods such as nuts, seeds or popcorn does not increase the risk for diverticulitis. In fact, a high-fiber diet, including fruit, vegetables, nuts and seeds, offers good nutrition and promotes regular bowel movements, both of which reduce the risk for diverticular disease.

• **Get vigorous exercise.** People who routinely run, hike, walk briskly, swim and/or do aerobics are significantly less at risk for diverticular problems than those who are sedentary—perhaps because vigorous exercise promotes circulation and helps fight constipation.

• **Try probiotics.** These "friendly" bacteria help keep colon inflammation at bay. Three times a week, eat eight ounces of plain yogurt with "live cultures" or take a probiotic supplement containing at least five billion units of *acidophilus* and 2.5 billion units of *bifidus*.

If you are diagnosed with diverticulitis...

• **Drink tea.** Most doctors recommend a liquid diet, including water, soup and juice, for three or four days. To reduce abdominal pain and speed healing, include tea made from peppermint, slippery elm and marshmallow root.

What to do: Blend equal parts by weight of each herb (chopped, shredded or powdered), and use two teaspoons of the mix per 10 ounces of boiling water. Have up to one quart of the tea daily.

• **Take Oregon grape root.** This herb has a sedating and antiseptic effect on the gastrointestinal tract and will ease cramping and reduce inflammation. Take 60 drops of Oregon grape root tincture in two ounces of water on an empty stomach, three times a day for up to seven days.

If you have abdominal pain and a fever of 101° or higher, rectal bleeding...or even mild abdominal pain that lasts for more than two days, see your doctor—each could signal an ailment that needs medical attention.

REPORT #25
Citrus Supplement Helps Stop Cancer From Spreading

Mark A. Stengler, NMD, naturopathic medical doctor in private practice, Encinitas, California...adjunct associate clinical professor at the National College of Natural Medicine, Portland, Oregon...author of *The Natural Physicians Healing Therapies* and coauthor of *Prescription for Natural Cures* (both from Bottom Line Books).

We usually think of the peels of oranges and grapefruit as good for compost heaps and garnish on foods and not much else. But research has found another use for a substance found in peels that is known as *pectin*—and it is at the root of a cancer therapy.

WHERE IT COMES FROM

Pectin is a compound found in the peel and pith (the white strands attached to the peel) of citrus fruits. It also is found in the peel and core of other fruits, such as apples. Even if you were to eat an orange peel, you wouldn't get any pectin that your body could use because in its natural state, its molecules are too large for us to digest. But researchers have found that when they break down pectin molecules into smaller sizes, it can be absorbed into the bloodstream.

Modified citrus pectin (MCP), which is what the over-the-counter supplement is called, has been found to stop the spread of cancer. (The word "modified" in this case means that the substance has been changed so that it can be absorbed by humans.) MCP is not meant to be used on its own as a cancer treatment, but it provides anticancer effects when used in conjunction with conventional cancer treatments such as chemotherapy. Its benefit is impressive because the spread (metastasis) of cancer from the original site to other parts of the body is the main cause of cancer-related death. MCP has been widely studied as a treatment for prostate and breast cancers and could help many other cancers.

HOW MCP WORKS

MCP prevents tumors from metastasizing by binding with a protein called galectin-3, a receptor molecule on the surface of cancer cells that usually carries out a number of cancer-promoting activities. One of galectin-3's most important functions involves helping cancer cells adhere to blood vessel walls and to other cancer cells, allowing the cells to colonize healthy body tissues. By binding with galectin-3, MCP blocks this adhesion process. MCP also blocks galectin-3's ability to stimulate the formation of blood vessels in new tumors, a process called angiogenesis that is essential to tumor growth...and it appears to encourage cancer-cell death (apoptosis) by interfering with signaling pathways related to cancer-cell proliferation and survival.

Galectin-3 also helps cancer cells survive chemotherapy treatment. MCP disrupts this, enabling chemotherapy to be more effective.

WHAT THE STUDIES SHOW

In a study published in *Integrative Cancer Therapies*, Columbia University researchers found that when prostate cancer cells were exposed to MCP in the laboratory, they died off. Its effect on androgen-independent prostate cancer (a prostate cancer in which cells do not depend on the androgen hormone for growth) is especially exciting, because there are not many effective treatments for this form of cancer, which tends to be aggressive.

A study conducted at Miami Children's Hospital (and funded by a supplement company that makes MCP) and published in *BMC Complementary and Alternative Medicine* found that MCP had a powerful effect on the immune system's ability to fight cancer, inducing a dose-dependent increase in cytotoxic T-cells and natural killer (NK) cells—two immune system components that attack and kill tumor cells. The study also found that the highest dose of MCP tested (800 micrograms per milliliter of blood in a lab sample, which has no exact equivalent in terms of an oral dose) increased NK cells' ability to destroy leukemia cancer cells by more than 50%. Some forms of chemotherapy fight galectin-3 molecules, too, but they also kill healthy cells. MCP is the first natural substance shown to fight galectin-3—and the hope is that with MCP the body's normal NK cell activity will work overtime to kill cancer cells while leaving healthy cells alone.

WHO SHOULD TAKE MCP

There's growing interest among holistic practitioners and some oncologists in MCP. One of MCP's most important features is that it is nontoxic. The only side effect is mild digestive upset. People can take MCP with other drugs—two hours apart is best, since MCP's fiber may hinder absorption of the other drugs. It also is safe for children.

MCP is a particularly good adjunct therapy for prostate and breast cancers, which have been the most studied. MCP's cancer-fighting ability also provides a protective benefit to cancer survivors and people with a family member (parent or sibling) who has had cancer.

One brand I like: PectaSol-C, a proprietary formulation developed and manufactured by EcoNugenics. PectaSol-C MCP can be purchased online at *www.econugenics.com*. Follow directions on the label.

REPORT #26
Raise Your IQ Nine Points in 10 Minutes

Arthur Winter, MD, neurosurgeon, and director, New Jersey Neurological Institute, Livingston. He is coauthor of *Brain Workout* (iUniverse) and *Build Your Brain Power* (St. Martin's).

Most people assume that everyone's mental capacities diminish with age. Fortunately, that's not true.

Recent studies show that cognitive decline doesn't occur in healthy older brains. With physical and mental stimulation, most can keep their cognitive abilities near maximum capacity as they age. Your brain continues to repair cell damage and form new neural networks throughout life. In fact, people who are active mentally can actually improve their scores on intelligence tests after age 60.

EXERCISES THAT WORK... EXERCISE YOUR BRAIN

Recent study: One study shows that sedentary individuals ages 55 to 70 who enlisted in a four-month aerobic exercise program did significantly better on neuropsychological tests than subjects who didn't perform aerobic exercise. Improved cognitive performance was attributed to increased blood flow to the brain.

Any aerobic exercise—walking, swimming, biking, etc.—also increases oxygenation of the brain and can improve memory as well as mood and speed of decision-making. Brisk walking for 30 minutes daily is adequate.

USE ALL YOUR SENSES

We gather information with the senses—and we are more likely to remember information when we use multiple senses.

Example: It's common to forget the name of someone you just met, partly because you only use one sense (hearing) when you're introduced. The next time you meet someone, bring more of your senses into play. Shake hands. Notice his/her scent and appearance. The more sensory details you accumulate, the more likely you are to store the name in memory.

Exercise: Sniff a bar of fragrant soap. Pay attention to how it looks and feels. Then read a paragraph from a book or magazine. Sniff the soap again. The next day, smell the soap again. You'll probably recall more of what you read than you would if you did not sniff the soap.

MEMORIZE SOMETHING DAILY

Memory is like a muscle—the more you use it, the stronger it becomes.

The brain stimulation that occurs while you're learning new material triggers an increase in the number of dendrites (sensors on nerves) as well as synapses (connections between the nerve cells).

Exercise: Learn one new word a day. Write it down on a notepad, and rehearse it in your mind a few times. The next day, write down a new word and review the one from the day before. Doing this daily will increase your vocabulary as well as your ability to retain new information.

Smart idea: Use a free online service, such as A.Word.A.Day. To subscribe, go to its Web site at *www.wordsmith.org/awad*. As an alternative, choose a word you don't know from your daily newspaper.

IMPROVE MEMORY WITH MUSIC

Music is a highly effective tool for improving brain function. The type of music is not important. Music reduces emotional and mental stress, both of which interfere with memory. Singing or playing a musical instrument stimulates the cerebellum and improves your ability to organize and recall new information.

A 1993 study of college students reported in *Nature* found that those who listened to Mozart for 10 minutes prior to a standardized intelligence test raised their scores to 119 (from 110 following silence).

Exercise: Practice a musical instrument or sing for 15 minutes several times daily. It doesn't matter if you can't carry a tune. Just the act of singing—accompanying words with rhythm—makes information easier to remember.

Helpful: If there's something specific you want to memorize—a phone number, address or shopping list—sing it out loud. This brings different parts of the brain into play and aids memorization.

MAKE ASSOCIATIONS

The brain is thought to store related information in discrete areas. When you recall a word from your long-term memory, there's a temporary increase in nerve activity in nearby locations. That's why the practice of association —linking certain words or concepts together —is an effective technique to practice to improve memory.

Exercise: Make a list of 20 simple words—dog, cat, bird, etc. Read the list of words once, then write down as many of them as you can remember. If you're good, you'll get about half of the words.

Then try the same thing while making associations for each word. The word "dog," for example, can be associated with a picture of a black Labrador or a pet you own. The more associations you make, the more words you'll remember.

PRACTICE SPEED

Using a timer or your watch, write down as many five-letter words as you can in two minutes. Repeat the exercise daily. If you want, practice with six-, seven- or eight-letter words. Your ability to recall all information will improve.

REPORT #27
Hope for Patients with Inoperable Tumors

Christopher Taylor Barry, MD, PhD, an associate professor of surgery at the University of Rochester Medical Center in Rochester, New York. A pioneer in IRE procedures, he is a member of the American Society of Transplant Surgeons and the Transplantation Society and has authored numerous professional articles in such journals as *Nature Biotechnology, Journal of Gastroenterology and Hepatology* and the *American Journal of Transplantation*. Dr. Barry reports that he has no financial interest in or special arrangements regarding the NanoKnife or AngioDynamics, its maker.

A "shocking" new treatment that some doctors believe offers hope to cancer patients with tumors that would have been inoperable in the past is now being used in 16 medical centers across the US.

Specially trained doctors can now use long, needlelike probes to deliver high-voltage bursts of electricity to tumors that are difficult to remove surgically. The minimally invasive procedure, known as irreversible electroporation (IRE), targets cancer cells that are then engulfed and removed by the body's immune system.

Intended benefits: Because IRE doesn't involve traditional "open" surgery, patients may experience little pain after the procedure. Some of them go home from the hospital the same day. Because the treatment generates little heat and the probes are precisely positioned through tiny incisions in the skin, there's a very low risk for damage to nearby nerves, blood vessels or organs.

Anecdotal evidence based on procedures that have been performed using IRE shows that this approach has proved successful in treating cancers of the liver, kidneys, pancreas, prostate and lungs. Thus far, the device has been used to perform about 300 procedures worldwide. In the future, it may be used for treating many different types of cancer, including malignancies of the breast and brain.

Important caveat: The device that is used to administer IRE, known as a NanoKnife, has not yet undergone randomized studies comparing it with other treatments—an important step in scientific research. Some doctors are concerned about the lack of clinical data.

MORE PRECISION, LESS PAIN?

Traditional cancer treatments, such as surgical removal or the destruction of cells with extreme heat (radiofrequency ablation) or cold (cryoablation), are somewhat imprecise, even in skilled hands. These procedures not only can damage some of the healthy tissue that surrounds the tumor, but also result in scar tissue that causes pain.

With IRE, it's now possible to attack tumors on an almost unthinkably small ("nano") scale. The electrical pulses punch very tiny holes in the walls of cancer cells and cause them to die. However, because of the lack of a head-to-head comparison with other techniques, it is unclear whether less pain is involved or precision is superior with IRE.

The NanoKnife has received FDA approval for soft-tissue ablation (removal) based on a regulatory provision that allows expedited approval without rigorous scientific testing. The approval was granted because the NanoKnife was deemed sufficiently similar to another medical device currently in use—one that is used to destroy tissue during heart operations.

Use of IRE is not intended to replace older cancer treatments. For now, it's mainly used for treating cancers that aren't readily removed with other procedures. It gives doctors an additional tool when treating tumors that are smaller than 5 cm (approximately 2 inches), are located in hard-to-reach areas or that can't be removed without a high risk of damaging nearby structures.

WHO MAY BENEFIT

The expected precision of IRE, and the fact that it may be less likely to produce scar tissue or damage healthy tissue than other procedures, means that there may be a lower risk for complications.

Example: Men who undergo prostate surgery often suffer from impotence or urinary incontinence because of damage to critical nerves. This damage has thus far been less likely with IRE.

In the future, IRE could become an important treatment for patients who can't withstand the trauma of major surgery. It's performed under general anesthesia but is much faster than traditional surgery and less physically taxing.

However, the anesthesia must be "deep" to keep patients completely immobile during the procedure. Otherwise, the probes could shift and potentially damage healthy tissue or fail to destroy portions of the tumor. Potential complications include inadvertent perforation of an organ or tissue, hemorrhage or infection.

HOW IT WORKS

Once the patient is anesthetized, a computed tomography (CT) scanner or ultrasound device is used to guide the placement of the probes. The doctor then uses a foot pedal to generate electrical bursts (each one lasting less than 100-millionths of a second) that kill the cancer cells within a particular area.

IRE treatment can cover an area that measures about 3 cm by 4 cm in less than four minutes. It's less effective for tumors larger than 5 cm. The standard treatment consists of a series of 90 electrical pulses.

Because this technology is so new, it is not yet widely available in the US. It's being used, and studied, in Europe and Australia.

Not all insurers cover the cost of treatment with IRE. Some cite a current lack of scientific evidence when declining claims for coverage.

Consult your physician for updates.

REPORT #28
The Nose Spray That "Eats Away" Alzheimer's Plaques

Howard L. Weiner, MD, principal investigator, Center for Neurologic Diseases, Brigham and Women's Hospital, Boston.
Journal of Clinical Investigation online

Researchers think they are close to devising a deceptively simple way to halt the progression of Alzheimer's disease—a vaccine in a nasal spray.

The vaccine, which so far has only been tested on mice, is a combination of two medications, Protollin and *glatiramer acetate* (Copaxone), which has already been approved to treat other conditions, including *multiple sclerosis* (MS).

The spray targets the abnormal buildup of *beta-amyloid plaque* in the brain. Many researchers believe that this amyloid accumulation is the main cause of Alzheimer's disease, although there is not yet enough evidence to support such a theory.

THE RESEARCH

The researchers sought to design a vaccine —administered via drops in the nose—that would initiate an amyloid-cleansing process by triggering the immune system without provoking antibody development, a problem that occurred in previous trials.

Study coauthor Howard L. Weiner, MD, principal investigator of the Center for Neurologic Diseases at Brigham and Women's Hospital, and his colleagues targeted microglial cells, which essentially eat away the amyloid buildup. The researchers tried to produce a vaccine that would stimulate these microglial cells into action.

Mice that had a similar amount of beta-amyloid plaque in their brains as what would be present in a human Alzheimer's patient, were given an initial four doses of the vaccine in the first week, followed by weekly doses for the next six weeks. The research team began monitoring the mice one week after vaccination for signs of disease, paralysis, limb weakness and fatigue.

Ultimately, brain tissue was dissected and examined for evidence of both amyloid quantity and any toxic side effects that might have developed in reaction to the vaccine.

The authors found that, overall, amyloid plaque levels in the vaccinated mice were reduced by 73%. None of the vaccinated mice showed any evidence of toxic side effects.

"I'm very hopeful [that this vaccine] could stimulate the immune system to reduce this buildup among people with early signs of Alzheimer's as well as for those in later stages of the disease," says Dr. Weiner.

THE NEXT STEP

Dr. Weiner and his team say they hope to begin small-scale testing of the Alzheimer's nasal spray vaccine in people following talks with the US Food and Drug Administration (FDA).

The human trial process will take time, the researchers point out, so a nasal Alzheimer's vaccine is, at best, several years away from clinical use.

Dr. Weiner notes that although there are a number of different research projects currently exploring the possibility of reducing beta-amyloid buildup in the brain, none has yet been shown to work in people. He also emphasizes that transitioning from animals to people is a tricky process that doesn't always work.

"But I'm very enthusiastic," he says. "I think it has a good chance of working and helping Alzheimer's patients—and even opening up a new avenue for developing a vaccine for MS."

For more information on Alzheimer's disease, visit the Web site of the Alzheimer's Association at *www.alz.org*.

REPORT #29
Some Drugs No Better Than Placebo for Alzheimer's Patients

Thomas Insel, MD, director, National Institute of Mental Health.

Gary J. Kennedy, MD, director of geriatric psychiatry, Montefiore Medical Center, New York, and former chairman of the Geriatric Mental Health Foundation, Bethesda, Maryland.

The New England Journal of Medicine

Antipsychotic drugs, which are commonly prescribed to treat psychosis, agitation and aggression in Alzheimer's patients, do benefit some patients, but the overall picture is bleak, recent research suggests.

Two of the drugs studied did seem to ease some symptoms, but the advantages were offset by the severity of the side effects.

MORE RESEARCH

"It's a call to arms to push the research forward much more quickly," conceded Thomas Insel, MD, director of the National Institute of Mental Health, which sponsored the study.

Newer antipsychotic medications are used widely for Alzheimer's patients, despite an absence of solid evidence of their efficacy.

"I hope this will highlight behavioral interventions which are effective though not perfect," said Gary J. Kennedy, MD, former chairman of the Geriatric Mental Health Foundation, in Bethesda, Maryland.

More than half of Alzheimer's patients experience delusions, hallucinations, aggression and agitation at some point in the progression of their disease. Traditional antipsychotics such as *haloperidol* have a lower risk of side effects than the newer agents, although both are thought to be equally effective.

SAFETY CONCERNS

Recently, however, concerns about safety have emerged with the second-generation drugs. Some studies have found an increased risk of cerebrovascular problems and even death.

This study involved 421 participants, all of whom had Alzheimer's disease along with psychosis, aggression or agitation. All participants also lived with a caregiver or in an assisted-living facility, not a nursing home, to give the study more relevance to a real-world setting.

THE STUDY

In the first phase of the study, participants were randomized to receive one of three of the newer antipsychotic medications—*olanzapine* (Zyprexa), *quetiapine* (Seroquel), *risperidone* (Risperdal)—or a placebo.

The investigators were mainly interested in how long patients could take the drugs before discontinuing. Regardless of whether they were taking an actual drug or a placebo, patients discontinued their medication, on average, after about eight weeks.

There were some outliers who benefited from treatment, including 26% to 32% of those taking the active medications who improved, compared with 21% of those on the placebo. Zyprexa and Risperdal seemed to perform better than Seroquel.

Much of this benefit, however, was counterbalanced by side effects such as sedation, confusion and weight gain. Some 15% to 24% of those taking an active medication discontinued their use because of side effects versus only 5% of those on the placebo.

Eighty-two percent of participants discontinued their medications in Phase I. These individuals are now participating in Phase 2 of the trial, in which they are randomized to one of the medications not previously taken or to *citalopram*, an antidepressant. The results of this phase are not yet available.

MONITORING THE RESULTS

For now, some patients may still benefit from this class of medication. "Even if they don't look like they're effective in a whole population of people, there are some people who will respond and who will be able to tolerate them, so we will probably want to continue to use these drugs with great care and close monitoring of side effects," Dr. Kennedy said.

Dr. Insel advocates the development of new and better drugs.

"In the future, treating psychosis [including schizophrenia] might be like treating hypertension," he said. "One medication isn't going to be the magic bullet. We need more than one, particularly in those with severe cases."

REPORT #30
"Old Age" Symptoms Could Really Be a Vitamin Deficiency

Sally M. Pacholok, RN, and Jeffrey J. Stuart, DO, co-authors of *Could It Be B-12?* (Linden). Ms. Pacholok has studied vitamin B-12 deficiency for more than 20 years. Dr. Stuart is a board-certified emergency medicine physician. Both are based in Rochester, Michigan.

Millions of Americans suffer tingling, numbness or pain in their hands or feet...dizziness...balance problems...depression...and/or memory loss because they are deficient in vitamin B-12, a nutrient that most of us—including many doctors—rarely think about. Low levels of vitamin B-12 can even raise the risk for heart disease and osteoporosis, according to research.

Good news: You can avoid the potentially serious complications of vitamin B-12 deficiency with simple, inexpensive treatment—if the problem is identified soon enough. Permanent damage can occur if the deficiency is not treated within a year of the development of symptoms.

What you need to know...

A KEY TO PROPER NERVE FUNCTION

Vitamin B-12 is needed to maintain the layers of tissue, known as the myelin sheath, that insulate each nerve cell. We need only a very tiny amount of the vitamin each day—2.4 micrograms (mcg).

The vitamin is abundant in meats (such as red meat, poultry and liver), shellfish, eggs and dairy products. Because vitamin B-12 is readily stored by the body (mainly in the liver), doctors have long assumed that deficiency is rare.

But a complex process must occur before vitamin B-12 can do its job. When it is consumed, the vitamin must be split from the proteins to which it is attached, carried into the small intestine and transported throughout the body with the help of other proteins.

If there is a problem—for example, a person takes a drug that interferes with vitamin B-12 absorption—a potentially dangerous deficiency can result. Among adults over age 65, up to 25% have been found in studies to have a clear B-12 deficiency (blood levels of less than 225).

THE TOLL OF B-12 DEFICIENCY

Many so-called symptoms of aging—both physical and mental—actually could be the result of B-12 deficiency. When a lack of this vitamin impairs the nervous system, a variety of problems can result, including weakness, dizziness and tremor—all of which can be mistaken for signs of neurological disorders, such as Parkinson's disease, multiple sclerosis, vertigo or neuropathy (nerve damage that causes pain or numbness).

A B-12 deficiency also can affect how you think, feel and act, resulting in irritability, apathy, confusion, forgetfulness—even serious depression, dementia, paranoia and/or hallucinations. Vitamin B-12 deficiency can lead to symptoms that are sometimes mistaken for Alzheimer's disease.

The cardiovascular system also can be affected. Vitamin B-12—along with vitamin B-6 and folic acid (another B vitamin)—plays a key role in the breakdown of homocysteine, a naturally occurring amino acid. Elevated levels of homocysteine damage blood vessels and promote the buildup of fatty deposits in the arteries (atherosclerosis) as well as abnormal blood clotting. Several studies have linked high blood levels of homocysteine to significantly increased risk for heart disease, heart attack, stroke and blood clots in the lungs and/or extremities.

The dangers of elevated homocysteine are widely known, but many doctors—cardiologists among them—simply prescribe high doses of folic acid to lower levels of the amino acid, ignoring the need to test for and possibly correct vitamin B-12 deficiency as well.

Also linked to B-12 deficiency…

• **Breast cancer.** A Johns Hopkins study of 390 women found that those with the lowest levels of B-12 were two to four times more likely to develop breast cancer than those with healthier levels.

• **Infections.** In another study, 30 older adults who had very low levels of B-12 produced fewer antibodies when vaccinated against pneumonia—leaving them with less protection against this potentially fatal infection than adults with adequate levels of B-12.

• **Osteoporosis.** Research shows that B-12 deficiency is linked to osteoporosis—in part, because B-12 is crucial to the function of osteoblasts (bone-forming cells).

ARE YOU AT RISK?

Aging is a primary risk factor for B-12 deficiency. That's because 30% to 40% of people over age 50 suffer from atrophic gastritis, which damages the stomach lining, markedly reducing production of the stomach acid needed to absorb vitamin B-12. Many older adults also fail to eat vitamin B-12-rich foods.

Another cause of B-12 deficiency is pernicious anemia—an autoimmune disorder in which the body does not produce a substance called intrinsic factor, which is necessary for the vitamin's absorption. Pernicious anemia is more common among people who have other autoimmune diseases, such as rheumatoid arthritis, lupus and thyroid disease, as well as type 1 diabetes.

It's now recognized that Crohn's disease (chronic inflammation of the intestinal wall) and celiac disease (intolerance to gluten, a protein found in wheat, barley and rye) can impede absorption of vitamin B-12. So can gastrointestinal surgery—particularly gastric bypass.

In addition, commonly used medications—such as the heartburn drugs known as proton pump inhibitors, including *omeprazole* (Prilosec) and *lansoprazole* (Prevacid)…and H2 blockers, including *ranitidine* (Zantac) and *famotidine* (Pepcid)…as well as the oral diabetes drug *metformin* (Glucophage, Glumetza)—can interfere with B-12 absorption.

Because vitamin B-12 is found only in animal products, strict vegetarians are at high risk for a deficiency. Some research shows that 80% of people who do not eat animal products and fail to take a B-12 supplement have a deficiency of the vitamin.

GET THE RIGHT TEST

When doctors order a complete blood count (CBC), among the abnormalities they look for is macrocytic anemia, a condition in which red blood cells are abnormally large. This can be a sign of vitamin B-12 deficiency. But in people who take supplements that contain folic acid—as do most multivitamins—blood test results may appear normal even when there is a vitamin B-12 deficiency. (Folic acid can "mask" such a deficiency.) A blood test that specifically measures B-12 levels also is available. However, this test is not always accurate—it has a wide "normal" range and can be inconsistent in its sensitivity.

The most sensitive B-12 test measures the amount of *methylmalonic acid* (MMA) in the urine. Because vitamin B-12 plays a key role in the production of MMA, results of this test can conclusively diagnose or rule out B-12 deficiency. Health insurance will pay for the test if the patient has symptoms of B-12 deficiency or is at high risk for deficiency.

BEST TREATMENT OPTIONS

If you have a B-12 deficiency, injections of 1,000 mcg—daily at first, then weekly, then monthly—are the most dependable solution, especially if neurologic symptoms are present. Sublingual (under-the-tongue) doses may be an alternative for some people. Ask your doctor. The MMA test should be repeated in three months to check the sublingual supplement's effectiveness.

If you have a B-12 deficiency, it's also wise to receive a homocysteine blood test before treatment to determine whether inadequate B-12 has raised your homocysteine levels, thus increasing your risk for vascular disease.

REPORT #31
How Nicotine Patches May Help Get Your Memory Back

Paul Newhouse, MD, director, Vanderbilt Center for Cognitive Medicine, Vanderbilt University School of Medicine, Nashville.

Jennifer Rusted, PhD, professor, experimental psychology, Sussex University, Brighton, UK.

Recent research suggests that the nicotine patches used by people trying to quit smoking could serve an unexpected purpose. They appear to counteract mild memory loss in older patients.

The research is preliminary and only involved a few dozen subjects.

There's also the matter of expense. While they're available over the counter, patches can cost several dollars a day.

Still, "nicotine treatment may be a way to improve people's symptoms and maybe extend their ability to do all of those cognitive things we need to do," said study author Paul Newhouse, MD, director of the Center for Cognitive Medicine at Vanderbilt University School of Medicine. "We're hoping to pursue this with a much larger group."

This isn't the first time researchers have tried to analyze connections between the brain and nicotine. In the 1980s, Dr. Newhouse and others discovered through autopsies that the brains of patients with Alzheimer's disease lacked certain "receptors" that help the brain's chemicals work properly, he said. Nicotine appears to stimulate these receptors, which revs up the system involved in attention, learning and memory skills.

However, it appears that nicotine isn't a huge help if someone already has a well-functioning ability to pay attention, he said.

STUDY DETAILS AND RESULTS

In the study, researchers recruited 74 non-smoking seniors with mild cognitive problems and watched what happened to 34 who received treatment with nicotine patches (15 milligrams a day) and 33 who got placebo patches for six months. Another seven didn't finish the study.

The people in the study weren't in bad enough shape to be diagnosed with Alzheimer's disease. However, they did have moments of memory loss that the people around them noticed, Dr. Newhouse said.

"They might repeat themselves, tell the same thing several times over or not remember something they've been told," he explained, "or make a mistake in calculations for their checkbook." Their losses in cognitive function were beyond those of normal aging, he added.

After testing cognition and memory at the start of the study and again at three and six months, the researchers found that those who used the real patches did better in terms of attention and memory, although the differences weren't huge and their doctors didn't notice them. The nicotine patch group regained 46% of their long-term memory loss, while the placebo patch group saw a 26% further decline in memory. Also, "people subjectively thought they were doing better," Dr. Newhouse said.

The only consistent side effect was weight loss, he said, and it's not clear if that stabilizes over time.

The participants who got the real patches didn't suffer withdrawal symptoms when they went off them, Dr. Newhouse said. "There's no worries about becoming dependent on it or wanting to take nicotine even though you shouldn't take it."

The patches seem to boost memory by affecting the brain's chemicals and allowing a person to pay attention more easily, he said. "Attention is necessary for memory to work."

However, Dr. Newhouse said he can't recommend the nicotine treatment for memory loss at this time. "If you want to think about it, discuss it with your physician," he said.

The study appeared in the journal *Neurology*. The researchers received federal funding for the research and the pharmaceutical company Pfizer contributed the nicotine patches.

EXPERT RESPONSE

Jennifer Rusted, PHD, a professor of experimental psychology at Sussex University in England, said the study was well done but it doesn't address the effectiveness of using nicotine patches in the long term. Also, Dr. Rusted said, there's debate about who should qualify as having mild cognitive problems in studies like this one.

As for the idea of taking nicotine patches to keep sharp mentally, she said that "realistically, the benefits even in this careful test were so small as to be indiscernible in the general scheme of daily activities. More important, there are many, many other ways of achieving much bigger improvements—exercise, diet, social and cognitive engagement and interaction."

For more about cognitive impairment, visit the Web site of the US National Library of Medicine at *http://www.nlm.nih.gov/medlineplus/mildcognitiveimpairment.html*.

REPORT #32
The "Clothing Cure" for Glaucoma

Robert Ritch, MD, professor of clinical ophthalmology, New York Medical College, Valhalla, and chief, Glaucoma Services, the New York Eye and Ear Infirmary, New York City.
British Journal of Ophthalmology

Ties that bind the neck may raise the risk of the eye disease glaucoma. So says a controversial study that found snug neckwear can increase intraocular pressure (IOP) in the eyes, possibly leading to glaucoma.

"If men wear tight neckties when their IOP is measured, it can raise their IOP," says Robert Ritch, MD, lead author of the study and a professor of clinical ophthalmology at New York Medical College.

DOUBLE TROUBLE

That double Windsor knot may be double trouble. If a person has moderate or severe glaucoma damage, the increase in IOP caused by a tight tie may make it worse. What's more, patients without glaucoma whose tight tie falsely increases IOP might end up being treated for glaucoma when they don't need to be. Although there are no reported cases of glaucoma being caused by a tight necktie, Dr. Ritch says it's theoretically possible.

Dr. Ritch became aware of the issue during his regular practice. "I noticed that some patients had tight neckties. When I loosened the neckties, their IOP would go down several points," he says.

To quantify his observation, Dr. Ritch and his colleagues looked at 20 healthy men and 20 men with open angle glaucoma, the most common form of the disease.

The researchers measured IOP first while the men weren't wearing neckties, then three minutes after they put on a tight necktie, and again three minutes after the tie was loosened.

Dr. Ritch's team found that in 70% of the healthy men, a tight necktie increased mean IOP, as it did in 60% of those with glaucoma.

Increases in IOP while wearing a tight necktie ranged from more than 2 mmHg to more than 4 mmHg (millimeters of mercury, a measure of pressure), compared with IOP readings when no ties were worn and after ties were loosened. This is a clinically important increase.

Dr. Ritch speculates that when a necktie exerts too much pressure on the jugular vein located in the neck, pressure is increased in the entire venous system, including in the eyes.

REPORT #33
Top Antihistamine Doesn't Work!

Karen Elizabeth Lasser, MD, MPH, assistant professor, department of medicine, Harvard Medical School, Boston, and Cambridge Health Alliance, Cambridge, Massachusetts. She was lead author of a study on the safety of new drugs published in *The Journal of the American Medical Association*.

A study published in *The Journal of the American Medical Association* examined all drugs approved by the US Food and Drug Administration (FDA) from 1975 to 1999. One drug in five was withdrawn from the market or required to have a "black-box" warning put on the package insert about serious risks.

During just one year of the study period, approximately 20 million Americans were given drugs that were later withdrawn.

The most common risks of the drugs were damage to the liver, heart and bone marrow and a variety of problems for pregnant women.

Self-defense: As long as other effective treatments are available, avoid any drug until it has been on the market for at least seven years. Approximately half of all problems with toxicity are discovered within that period.

Drugs to avoid—and better alternatives...

ALLERGY

•***Desloratadine* (Clarinex).** Introduced to the market in 2002, this antihistamine is essentially the same as the older drug *loratadine* (Claritin), which is broken down in the body into desloratadine. The manufacturer simply got a patent for the chemical by-product.

Drawbacks: There's no evidence that desloratadine is clinically different from loratadine. Neither is particularly effective.

In fact, when the manufacturer submitted four clinical trials to the FDA comparing doses of desloratadine with a placebo, only two of the studies found the drug to be effective.

Better choice: Over-the-counter (OTC) antihistamines, such as *chlorpheniramine* (Chlor-Trimeton) or *diphenhydramine* (Benadryl). They are not only less expensive but they are usually more effective. However, some people find them too sedating.

As an alternative, ask your doctor about prescription nasal steroids, such as *flunisolide* (Nasalide) or *beclomethasone* (Vancenase). They quickly ease congestion without the grogginess that is sometimes caused by antihistamines.

HEARTBURN

•***Esomeprazole* (Nexium).** Introduced in 2001, esomeprazole is the fifth member of the proton pump inhibitor class of drugs used for gastroesophageal reflux disease (heartburn) and for duodenal ulcers that don't respond to antacids or H-2 blockers, such as *cimetidine* (Tagamet).

Drawbacks: An FDA evaluation suggests that esomeprazole is no better than *omeprazole* (Prilosec), an older OTC proton pump inhibitor that has a known safety record.

Better choice: People who have heartburn can choose among many drugs—Prilosec, Tagamet, antacids, etc.—that have been on the market for a long time and are known to be safe.

Non-drug treatments, such as not lying down after meals and avoiding foods known to cause heartburn, are often all that's needed.

INSOMNIA

•***Zaleplon* (Sonata).** Introduced in 1999, zaleplon was designed to help insomnia patients fall asleep without the residual grogginess that is so common with other sleeping pills. Zaleplon is quickly eliminated from the body, so you can potentially take it late at night or early in the morning and still be fully alert when you get up.

Drawbacks: It's less potent than older sleeping pills, such as *triazolam* (Halcion), *temazepam* (Restoril) and *flurazepam* (Dalmane).

Compared with a placebo, zaleplon decreases the time it takes to fall asleep by only eight to 20 minutes. It has a high risk for addiction when taken for more than several weeks.

Zaleplon also has potentially serious interactions, such as excessive drowsiness, when it is taken with other drugs, including antihistamines and anti-ulcer medications.

Better choice: Behavioral and lifestyle adjustments, such as reducing caffeine intake and practicing yoga, are safer for treating insomnia.

For patients who need help for a few nights, older drugs such as *zolpidem* (Ambien) or *oxazepam* (Serax) can be effective.

REPORT #34
Protect the Family from The Flu—No Vaccine Needed

Mark A. Stengler, NMD, naturopathic medical doctor and leading authority on the practice of alternative and integrated medicine. Dr. Stengler is author of the *Health Revelations* newsletter, author of *The Natural Physician's Healing Therapies* (Bottom Line Books), founder and medical director of the Stengler Center for Integrative Medicine in Encinitas, California, and adjunct associate clinical professor at the National College of Natural Medicine in Portland, Oregon. http://markstengler.com

No one knows what the new flu season will bring. I have developed a flu-prevention protocol that can lower your risk of contracting any of the flu strains. It also can reduce the severity of your illness if you do get sick.

First question: When my patients ask me if they should get the flu vaccine I tell them that my family and I, and many of my patients, are not planning to. And I don't recommend that other healthy people get it either. I have several concerns about flu vaccines—namely, that we don't know the long-term impact of using them...many contain a mercury-based preservative (mercury is known to suppress the immune system)...and some people develop a flulike illness after receiving the vaccine. The truth is that the vaccines' effectiveness is, at best, hit or miss. However, the regular seasonal flu vaccine (mercury-free is best) should be considered for those who are over age 65... suffer from chronic pulmonary or cardiovascular disease...are nursing home residents... have a weakened immune system from chronic disease, such as cancer...or are pregnant.

What everyone needs when combating the flu is a strong immune system. The natural therapies I recommend can enhance and fine-tune your immune system. People who take these supplements, eat a healthful diet, get some exercise and sleep for at least seven hours a night have more protection against the flu than they would get from the flu vaccine.

MY FLU-PROTECTION PROTOCOL

Begin this protection protocol in November—and continue it through April.

•**Influenzinum.** At the heart of my flu-protection program is Influenzinum, a homeopathic remedy that is a safe alternative to conventional flu shots. I have recommended it to my patients for 15 years—with good results. Influenzinum has been prescribed by homeopathic physicians for the last 150 years and is reported to have protected people against the Spanish flu of 1918. It contains a homeopathic preparation of the flu virus that is made each year based on the predicted flu strains. In 1998, the French Society of Homeopathy concluded a 10-year survey of 23 homeopathic doctors and their use of Influenzinum for flu prevention in 453 patients.

Result: Only 10% of those who took it got the flu.

Action plan: Follow label instructions. Adults and children (age six and older) should take one dose (at least two pellets or a small vial of several pellets) of a 9C potency once a week for four weeks...wait a month...and then take a fifth dose. (For infants starting as young as one day old, crush one pellet and place on the tongue.) Many health-food stores carry Influenzinum. One good brand is made by Homeopathic Educational Services (800-359-9051, *www.homeopathic.com*).

- **Vitamin D.** Studies show that vitamin D protects against upper respiratory infections and can enhance the body's production of *cathelicidin*, a germ-killing compound.

Action plan: Adults and teenagers take 2,000 international units (IU) of vitamin D-3 daily and children 1,000 IU. Increase this amount to 5,000 IU daily for adults and 2,000 IU for children during peak flu season (January through March).

- **N-acetylcysteine (NAC).** Italian researchers found that seniors who took this antioxidant had virtually no flu symptoms, even though testing showed that they were infected, whereas people taking placebos in the same study suffered the brunt of flu symptoms. Research supports NAC's pulmonary benefits.

Action plan: Adults and teenagers take 1,000 milligrams (mg) of NAC daily and children (age six to 12 years old) take 500 mg daily. At the first sign of symptoms, immediately increase the amount to 4,000 mg daily (1,500 mg daily for children) and continue until symptoms are gone.

IF YOU DO GET THE FLU

To treat the flu, use the remedies described here and add the ones below to your regimen. Take them for as long as symptoms last, unless otherwise indicated. These supplements are safe, in these amounts, for everyone.

Take for the first two days only...

- **Oscillococcinum.** This homeopathic remedy is made from animal organ–derived ingredients that provide natural immunity to the flu virus. It can ease flu symptoms if taken within 48 hours after they start.

Action plan: Follow label directions for use, beginning on the first day of a cold or flu.

Take for as long as symptoms last...

- **Lomatium.** This herbal remedy (*Lomatium dissectum*) was used by Native Americans to treat respiratory infections. It has well-documented antimicrobial properties.

Action plan: Look for an alcohol- or glycerin-based tincture of lomatium. Follow label directions for use.

Note: Lomatium may amplify the effect of blood-thinning medications, so check with your doctor first if you are taking warfarin or any other blood-thinning medication. If you develop a rash or nausea, stop taking it.

- **Elderberry** (*Sambucus nigra L.*) Studies show that it significantly improves flu symptoms within two to four days.

Action plan: My favorite elderberry product is Sambucol syrup, available at drugstores (*www.sambucolusa.com* for a store locator). Follow label directions.

REPORT #35
Never Use a Spoon to Measure Meds

Mayo Clinic study participants were asked to pour one teaspoon of cold medicine into different-sized kitchen spoons. They either under- or overpoured mainly because kitchen spoons hold more or less than an official-sized teaspoon.

Best: Use a measuring cap or a dosing spoon when administering medication.

Mark A. Stengler, NMD, naturopathic medical doctor and leading authority on the practice of alternative and integrated medicine. Dr. Stengler is author of the *Health Revelations* newsletter, author of *The Natural Physician's Healing Therapies* (Bottom Line Books), founder and medical director of the Stengler Center for Integrative Medicine in Encinitas, California, and adjunct associate clinical professor at the National College of Natural Medicine in Portland, Oregon. *http://markstengler.com*

REPORT #36
Don't Drink the Water

Mark A. Stengler, NMD, naturopathic medical doctor and leading authority on the practice of alternative and integrated medicine. Dr. Stengler is author of the *Health Revelations* newsletter, author of *The Natural Physician's Healing Therapies* (Bottom Line Books), founder and medical director of the Stengler Center for Integrative Medicine in Encinitas, California, and adjunct associate clinical professor at the National College of Natural Medicine in Portland, Oregon. *http://markstengler.com*

Have you ever wondered why there is a warning on the labels of toothpastes? It tells users to keep the product away from children and to seek medical attention if more than the recommended amount for brushing is swallowed.

Reason: Toothpaste contains fluoride.

For years, this chemical has been added to our water to reduce the occurrence of dental cavities—but unbelievably, the newest evidence shows that fluoridated water does not protect against cavities. In fact, it turns out that we don't need fluoride to protect our teeth at all.

Dentists advise that children use toothpaste that contains fluoride—and yet we keep all kinds of other medications and dangerous products away from children. But is toothpaste as dangerous? Yes. The average tube of toothpaste contains enough fluoride to kill a child. And how safe is a glass of fluoridated tap water?

Fluoride occurs naturally in soil, water and some plants. It also is a by-product of phosphate fertilizer production and is an industrial waste product of the aluminum smelting industry. The FDA maintains that fluoride is a drug. It's also known to be a highly toxic substance, even more toxic than lead. Once used as rat poison, it can cause serious health problems when ingested in unsafe amounts, including weak bones, hormone disruption and neurological damage.

And the truth is—fluoride is everywhere. It's not only in dental-hygiene products but also still in our water supply. It's been there since the 1940s, when extensive tooth decay was common across the US. In 1999, the Centers for Disease Control and Prevention (CDC) called water fluoridation one of the 10 greatest public health achievements of the 20th century.

Fast forward to 2013...and we are at risk for health problems because we are overexposed to fluoride. It is even in a number of products that our families consume (either when we add in fluoridated water or when the products themselves are made with fluoridated water), such as baby formula, processed cereals, juice, soda, tea, wine and beer. *What you need to know to protect yourself...*

FLUORIDE IN TAP WATER

It's not only the natural medicine community that is alarmed. In 2011, for the first time in about 50 years, the US Department of Health and Human Services (HHS) announced that there was too much fluoride in the US water supply and recommended reducing the amount of fluoride added to water to 0.7 parts per million (ppm) everywhere. The limit had previously been 0.7 ppm in warm climates where people drink a lot of water to 1.2 ppm in cooler climates (where people presumably drink less).

FLUORIDE CAUSES HEALTH PROBLEMS

When you ingest fluoride, about half is excreted by the kidneys. The rest is stored in your bones and teeth, where it does the opposite of what it is supposed to do—it causes damage. According to the CDC, 41% of American adolescents now have dental *fluorosis,* an increase from 23% in 1987. This disfigurement of tooth enamel in teeth, which can range from white patches to brown mottling, typically occurs before age eight (when permanent teeth are all formed). This very high rate of fluorosis is thought to be caused by fluoride intake during childhood, from drinking fluoridated water (including commercial drinks made with fluoridated water) and swallowing toothpaste with fluoride.

In addition to fluorosis, fluoride causes other health problems...

•**Fluoride decreases bone strength.** A 2010 *Journal of Dental Research* study found that bone strength in animals decreases with increased levels of fluoride in bones. HHS also has noted that excess fluoride can result in bone fractures and skeletal fluorosis, a crippling condition.

•**Fluoride impairs brain function in children.** A 2008 systematic review published in *Biological Trace Element Research* found that children in China who live in an area with fluoridated water have five times greater risk for a lower IQ than children who live in a nonfluoridated or slightly fluoridated area. The water was fluoridated at a level of 2.47 milligrams per liter (mg/L), three times the US safe level. (Note that 1 ppm equals 1 mg/L.)

•**Fluoride upsets cardiac function.** Increased fluoride can result in abnormal calcification of cardiac tissue. This can impair cardiac function in animals, say researchers from Agricultural University Wageningen in the Netherlands, whose study was published in *Biological Trace Element Research*.

•**Fluoride interferes with cell metabolism.** Research published in *Toxicology Letters* in 2010 points to chronic fluoride exposure as a possible cause of oxidative stress, which results in inflammation throughout the body.

In addition, in 2006, the National Research Council (NRC) reviewed EPA water-safety standards. The NRC found that excessive fluoride intake was associated with hormone disruption, impaired thyroid function, increased free radical activity in the brain (potentially contributing to dementia) and abnormal insulin response.

Population studies show that people who live in communities that fluoridate their water have no fewer cavities, on average, than people in communities without fluoridated water. While it's true that the US has experienced dramatic declines in cavities and tooth decay over the past 50 years, the same holds true for people in Europe, where many countries discontinued the practice of water fluoridation starting in the 1970s. It is believed that cavities have decreased despite water fluoridation cessation because of better oral hygiene.

MINIMIZE YOUR FLUORIDE INTAKE

Water fluoridation is an unsafe practice that should be stopped. If you live in the US, there's a 70% chance that your tap water is fluoridated. Since water fluoridation is left up to individual states and municipalities, practices vary from town to town.

Examples: New York City, Minneapolis and Chicago currently maintain a water fluoride content of 1 mg/L. To check the fluoride content of your water, contact your local water utility or visit *http://apps.nccd.cdc.gov/mwf/index.asp*. You can join the growing number of people who are letting their local government agencies know about the health concerns of fluoridated water.

To further protect yourself…

•**Drink spring water.** It usually contains less than 0.1 ppm of fluoride.

•**Use a water filter.** One of the best types of filters for removing fluoride is the reverse-osmosis filter, available at appliance stores for $300 to $400. Many household filters, such as Brita and Pur, do not eliminate fluoride.

AVOIDING FLUORIDE IN DENTAL PRODUCTS

The concentration of fluoride in many commercially made toothpastes is high—about 1,000 ppm to 1,500 ppm. Even when you don't swallow fluoridated toothpaste, some fluoride is absorbed by the body and goes into the bloodstream. I'm convinced that there is no benefit from any kind of topical application of fluoride—whether it's toothpaste, mouthwash or even a onetime fluoride treatment from the dentist. Both children and adults should not use fluoride treatment or supplements of any kind.

Switch to a toothpaste that doesn't include fluoride—and that does contain only natural ingredients. Make sure these include xylitol, a compound derived from plant fibers that is known to prevent cavities. Many such toothpastes are available at health-food stores. Also, work with a holistic dentist to ensure dental health.

REPORT #37
Deadly Virus Found in Florida

Dozens of cases of dengue fever have been reported in South Florida. The potentially deadly viral illness is transmitted by the Aedes mosquito. Symptoms include high fever, severe headache, rash and pain in bones and joints. Treatment includes bed rest, pain medicines and fluid replacement. There is no vaccine to prevent dengue fever. When in Florida, stay indoors at times when Aedes mosquitoes are most likely to bite—at dawn and dusk. If you must go out, apply a repellent containing the compound DEET to the skin and one containing permethrin to clothing, as directed. Stay away from stagnant water.

Carol L. De Rosa, RN, senior vice president of clinical services, Passport Health, provider of travel medicine services and vaccines, Baltimore. *www.passporthealthusa.com*

REPORT #38
Cold Sores May Be Linked to Alzheimer's Disease

Research has shown that a herpes simplex infection—the virus that causes cold sores—increases the amount of amyloid precursor protein, the parent protein of the plaque associated with Alzheimer's disease.

Self-defense: Treat cold sores quickly with an antiviral agent to minimize the amount of time that the virus remains active.

Elaine Bearer, MD, PhD, Harvey Family Professor and vice-chair for research, departments of pathology and neurosurgery, University of New Mexico School of Medicine, Albuquerque, and principal investigator in a study published in *PLoS One.*

REPORT #39
A New Treatment May Eliminate Tinnitus

Researchers were able to eliminate tinnitus (persistent ringing in the ears) in rats by stimulating the vagus nerve in the back of the neck while playing a variety of tones.

Theory: The technique releases chemicals that encourage changes in the brain and resets the brain's auditory system, eliminating tinnitus.

Michael Kilgard, PhD, professor, School of Behavioral and Brain Sciences, University of Texas, Dallas, and leader of the animal study published in the online edition of *Nature.*

REPORT #40
Beans Lower Blood Sugar

In a recent study, diabetics who ate one-half cup of beans a day—garbanzo, black, white, pinto or kidney beans—had significantly lower fasting glucose, insulin and hemoglobin A1C, a marker of long-term glucose control. When eaten as a regular part of a high-fiber, low-glycemic-index diet, beans lower hemoglobin A1C by an average of 0.48%, which lies at the lower level of effectiveness for medications such as *metformin* (Glucophage).

Cyril Kendall, PhD, research scientists, Department of Nutritional Sciences, University of Toronto, and the Clinical Nutrition and Risk Factor Modification Centre, St. Michael's Hospital, Toronto, and leader of research analyzing 41 trials regarding the effects of beans on blood sugar levels, published in *Diabetologia.*

REPORT #41
Yes, You Can Prevent Diabetes Complications

Neal D. Barnard, MD, adjunct associate professor of medicine at George Washington University School of Medicine and president of the nonprofit Physicians Committee for Responsible Medicine, a Washington, DC–based group that promotes preventive medicine and higher standards of effectiveness and ethics in research. He is author of *Dr. Neal Barnard's Program for Reversing Diabetes* (Rodale). www.nealbarnard.org

Diabetes is a slow and often "silent" disease. Most people who have it feel fine initially. By the time they develop symptoms, years of elevated blood sugar (glucose) have already caused widespread damage and complications, including cardiovascular disease, nerve damage and kidney disease.

Unfortunately, complications from diabetes can shorten life expectancy by about a decade.

Good news: Most people can reduce or eliminate these complications by maintaining optimal glucose control.

Here, the dangerous complications of diabetes and how to control them...

PERIPHERAL NEUROPATHY

Excess blood sugar can damage capillaries—tiny blood vessels—in the fingers, legs and/or feet. A lack of circulation to nerves can cause neuropathy, which can be painful and produce sensations of numbness, tingling and burning.

Important finding: One of my colleagues had his patients with neuropathy eat a low-fat, vegan diet (no animal foods or dairy products) and take a daily 30-minute walk. In 17 out of 21 patients, leg pain stopped completely—the remaining four had partial relief.

Many patients with neuropathy eventually lose all sensation in the extremities. This is dangerous because small injuries, such as cuts or an ingrown nail, for example, won't be noticed and can progress to serious infections and tissue damage—and, in some cases, require amputation. *What to do...*

•**Exercise daily.** It helps with weight loss and glucose control, which help reduce capillary damage and may reduce pain from neuropathy.

•**Check your feet every day.** Look for abrasions, cuts and blisters. See a doctor if an injury isn't healing.

Also, ask your doctor to examine your feet two to four times a year. Most doctors don't do this routinely.

Helpful: Take off your shoes and socks while you're waiting in the examination room. This makes it impossible for the doctor to ignore your feet.

EYE DAMAGE

Diabetes is the leading cause of blindness in American adults. High blood sugar can lead to glaucoma, resulting in optic nerve damage, which causes loss of vision. It also can damage the retinas (retinopathy) or the lenses of the eyes (cataracts). *What to do...*

•**Avoid dairy.** Many people lack the enzyme needed to metabolize galactose, a sugar that is released when the lactose in dairy is digested. This can lead to lens damage and cataracts.

•**Eat more produce.** The antioxidants in fresh fruits and vegetables, such as vitamin C, lutein and zeaxanthin, appear to have a stabilizing effect on the retina and can reduce the risk for cataracts and other eye diseases.

I do not recommend supplements for eye health because natural foods provide large amounts of these nutrients. It's likely that the combination of nutrients in foods, rather than single-source nutrients, offer the most protection.

PERIODONTAL DISEASE

Doctors have known for a long time that patients with diabetes have a high risk for periodontal disease, a chronic bacterial infection of the gums that can lead to tooth loss.

Recent finding: A review of research by the Cochrane Database of Systematic Reviews found that people with diabetes who were treated for periodontal disease achieved better blood sugar control, indicating that periodontal disease is both caused by and causes higher blood sugar. Periodontal treatment includes regular scaling, the removal of bacteria and inflammatory material from beneath the gums. *What to do…*

•**See your dentist four times a year.** The usual twice-a-year schedule might not be enough for people with diabetes.

•**Eat less sugar.** This is important for everyone, but more so for those with diabetes and periodontal disease. A high-sugar diet makes it easier for bacteria to proliferate.

•**Floss and brush your teeth after every meal**—not just once or twice a day.

HEART DISEASE

Most people in the US have some degree of atherosclerosis, plaque buildup in the arteries that increases the risk for heart attack. The risk for heart disease is much higher in people with diabetes, particularly when atherosclerosis is accompanied by hypertension and kidney disease.

Recent finding: People with diabetes who eat a typical American diet tend to accumulate *intramyocellular lipids,* tiny bits of fat inside muscle cells. This fat inhibits the ability of cells to respond to insulin, which leads to elevated blood sugar. *What to do…*

•**Avoid animal products and added fats.** Research by Dean Ornish, MD, showed that people who get no more than about 10% of total calories from fat (preferably unsaturated) can reverse blockages in the arteries. (Traditional diabetes diets allow up to 35% of calories from fat.)

•**Reduce cholesterol.** It's one of the best ways to reduce cardiovascular risks.

Helpful: Foods that are high in soluble fiber, such as oatmeal, fruits, whole grains and beans. People who eat beans regularly have average cholesterol readings that are about 7% lower than those who don't eat beans.

•**Reduce blood pressure.** The same strategies that reduce cholesterol and arterial blockages also reduce blood pressure.

KIDNEY DISEASE

The filtering units of the kidneys, or nephrons, consist of millions of small blood vessels that frequently are damaged by diabetes. Extensive damage can lead to kidney failure and the need for a transplant. *What to do…*

•**Give up animal protein.** The sulfur-containing amino acids in meats and eggs are harder for the nephrons to process than the proteins from plant foods. People with diabetes who switch to a vegetarian diet have a lower risk of developing kidney disease.

•**Maintain healthy blood pressure.** Uncontrolled hypertension is a leading cause of kidney failure. The same low-fat, plant-based diet that reduces glucose and cholesterol also is effective for lowering blood pressure.

ALZHEIMER'S DISEASE

A Japanese study reported in *Neurology* found that patients with type 2 diabetes or resistance to insulin were more likely to develop brain plaques, clusters of abnormal proteins that occur in those with Alzheimer's disease.

It's not yet clear whether diabetes increases the risk of getting Alzheimer's or there's an underlying process that causes both conditions. *What to do…*

•**Avoid meat.** Many studies have shown that people who eat diets that are high in meat, fat and cholesterol are more likely to develop Alzheimer's disease than those who eat a healthier diet. It's possible that the heme iron in meats is more likely than the non-heme iron in plant foods to be associated with brain plaques.

REPORT #42
Diabetic Kidney Disease Supplement May Help

Mahmood S. Mozaffari, PhD, DMD, professor and interim chairman, department of oral biology, Medical College of Georgia, Augusta.

Kidney disease is more common than you might guess—for instance, about 40% of people with diabetes will get kidney damage, or nephropathy, so news of a treatment that might ease the condition is certainly welcome. Here's that news: A study has found that the mineral supplement chromium picolinate may be helpful in staving off diabetic kidney disease, which is caused when high blood sugar destroys the small blood vessels of the kidneys. With 17.9 million Americans suffering from diabetes, this is good news indeed.

First, a tiny bit of background on diabetic nephropathy. If it is left untreated, the kidneys won't filter waste from the blood efficiently, which will eventually lead to kidney failure and the need for dialysis. Conventional preventive advice for this condition focuses on regular exercise, known to improve insulin sensitivity... keeping blood glucose levels down...controlling blood pressure, since high blood pressure can also damage the kidney's blood vessels... keeping cholesterol down...eating a low-fat diet... limiting salt and protein...and not smoking. But diabetic kidney disease continues to cause morbidity and mortality, thus indicating the need for other measures.

CAN CHROMIUM PICOLINATE HELP?

In research presented at a recent Conference of the American Physiological Society, Mahmood Mozaffari, PhD, DMD, a professor at the Medical College of Georgia, and his colleague Babak Baban, PhD, tested the effectiveness and safety of the supplement chromium picolinate for people at risk for diabetic nephropathy. Chromium picolinate has been suggested to help enhance the action of insulin and control glucose levels in patients with diabetes, especially type 2.

The researchers compared three groups of mice—one healthy group and two groups that were genetically engineered for obesity and diabetes (two conditions that often coexist). For six months, the healthy mice and one group of diabetic mice were fed a regular rodent diet. The other group of diabetic mice was fed a diet enriched with chromium picolinate. The researchers measured blood glucose levels and urinary albumin, a marker for kidney damage. As expected, they found that the untreated diabetic mice excreted nearly 10 times more albumin (an indication of kidney disease) than the healthy mice...but, the diabetic mice eating the chromium picolinate-enriched diet excreted only about half as much albumin as the untreated diabetic mice. In addition, kidney tissue samples showed changes suggestive of less inflammation in the treated diabetic group than in the untreated group. However, chromium picolinate treatment resulted in only a mild improvement in glucose control. Thus the researchers believe that effects other than sugar control may underlie the impact of the chromium picolinate in reducing biomarkers of inflammation in the kidney.

Chromium picolinate supplements are sold at most pharmacies or online in doses from 200 mcg to 800 mcg.

SHOULD YOU TRY IT?

While you can get some of the chromium you need from foods—such as broccoli, beef, chicken, turkey, red wine, wheat germ, eggs, black pepper and molasses or the probiotic brewer's yeast—dietary chromium is poorly absorbed from the gut.

Dr. Mozaffari cautions that this promising animal study must be substantiated in other studies including human clinical trials, so he is not yet advocating that people with diabetes should take chromium picolinate to help reduce the impact of diabetic nephropathy. And you definitely shouldn't be taking supplemental chromium if you are on medication for your diabetes, including if you're taking insulin, *metformin* (Glucophage) or *glyburide* (Diabeta), as it will affect the way your body reacts to the drugs...or if you take NSAIDs and antacids.

REPORT #43
Topical Gel Beats Bladder Problems

Gelnique, the first topical gel to treat overactive bladder (loss of bladder control), has been approved by the FDA. The gel is applied once daily to the thigh, abdomen, upper arm or shoulder. In a 12-week study of 789 women and men with overactive bladder, Gelnique decreased incontinence episodes by 10% and urination frequency by 6%, compared with a placebo. Gelnique is not metabolized by the liver, thus reducing side effects. Patients with urinary retention (inability to pass urine) or gastric retention (intestinal blockage) or uncontrolled narrow-angle glaucoma should not use Gelnique.

Christine P. Nguyen, MD, medical officer, division of reproductive and urological products, Center for Drug Evaluation and Research, FDA, Silver Spring, Maryland.

REPORT #44
Newer Blood Thinner Dangerous for Trauma Patients

Bryan Cotton, MD, trauma surgeon and intensivist, Memorial Hermann Hospital and University of Texas Health Science Center, Houston.

Lisandro Irizarry, MD, chair of emergency medicine, Brooklyn Hospital Center, New York City.

Jack Ansell, MD, chairman, department of medicine, Lenox Hill Hospital, New York City.

Statement, Boehringer Ingelheim US, Ridgefield, Connecticut.

New England Journal of Medicine

A new blood thinner touted for its convenience and low maintenance may have hidden problems that could threaten the lives of certain patients, a report suggests.

A letter to the editor of *The New England Journal of Medicine* reports severe bleeding complications among trauma patients on the anti-clotting medicine *dabigatran etexilate (Pradaxa)*.

In one case, a patient died, the letter said.

"We have noted on multiple occasions patients who have 'bleeding out' from Pradaxa and our hands are tied," said Bryan Cotton, MD, lead letter author and a trauma surgeon with the University of Texas Health Science Center at Memorial Hermann Hospital in Houston.

REVERSIBILITY A PROBLEM FOR PRADAXA

The main problem, Dr. Cotton said, is that there's no real way to reverse the anti-clotting effect of the drug, unlike older agents such as *warfarin*.

The only way to reverse Pradaxa is with emergency dialysis but, said Dr. Cotton, "in a patient bleeding to death, that's not really a practical or pragmatic option."

BACKGROUND

Warfarin (Coumadin, Jantoven) has been the mainstay of blood-thinning medications to manage heart and stroke patients for decades.

But the drug is notoriously difficult to manage, requiring frequent lab tests and having interactions with multiple foods and other medications. Its one big advantage, however, is that its blood-thinning properties are easily reversible when needed.

Enter the new, easier-to-use blood thinner, Pradaxa, first approved by the US Food and Drug Administration in late 2010 for use in patients with atrial fibrillation, a common and dangerous form of irregular heartbeat.

"There is an advantage over warfarin in many ways because of the simplicity and ease of management," said Jack Ansell, MD, chairman of the department of medicine at Lenox Hill Hospital in New York City. "There are very few interactions with other drugs or foods." On the other hand, he says, "warfarin is relatively easy to reverse."

OTHER ISSUES

Pradaxa also has other problems in addition to the irreversibility, the letter said, namely that there are no readily available tests to assess how well it's working or not working.

"You can't really check the labs. There's no easy, cheap, readily available lab test," Dr. Cotton noted.

The information provided in the letter, said Lisandro Irizarry, MD, chair of emergency medicine at the Brooklyn Hospital Center in New York City, is "incredibly useful and incredibly timely."

"Although this medication provides enhanced quality of life, it does have a significant impact on how we manage patients because there's no way to reverse it and no way to measure how thin the blood is," he said.

Dr. Cotton and his coauthors urged the US Food and Drug Administration (FDA) to support more trials to assess the potentially wide-ranging effects of the drug.

"We absolutely understand that it's a lot better for patients from a convenience standpoint…but when something goes wrong, it can go wrong very badly," Dr. Cotton said.

SAFETY A PRIORITY, SAYS MANUFACTURER

In a statement, Pradaxa's maker, Boehringer Ingelheim, confirmed that, "At this time, there is no reversal agent available" for the blood thinner. The company says that dialysis can lead to "the removal of about 60% of the drug over two to three hours; however, data supporting this approach are limited."

In the meantime, "Patient safety is our top priority and we frequently communicate with the FDA and regulatory agencies around the world to ensure they have the most up-to-date information regarding the safety profile of Pradaxa," the company said. "All treatment decisions should be made on an individual basis between patients and their health care providers and should take into consideration the overall benefits and risks associated with various treatment options."

Pradaxa is not the only new-generation blood thinner to be approved recently—the anti-clotting drug *ticagrelor* (Brilinta) gained FDA approval for use in heart patients this past summer. However, according to Dr. Ansell, there is no "reversibility" problem with Brilinta.

info The Web site of the National Library of Medicine has more on blood thinners. Visit *www.nlm.nih.gov/medlineplus/bloodthinners.html*.

REPORT #45
The 15-Minute Heart Cure

John M. Kennedy, MD, medical director of preventive cardiology and wellness at Marina Del Rey Hospital, California. He is a clinical associate professor at Harbor-UCLA Medical Center and is on the board of directors for the American Heart Association. He is author, with Jason Jennings, of *The 15 Minute Heart Cure: The Natural Way to Release Stress and Heal Your Heart in Just Minutes a Day* (Wiley). *www.the15minuteheartcure.com*

Most people know that smoking, high cholesterol and high blood pressure are among the main risk factors for heart disease. Few of us realize that daily stress is another key risk factor. It can damage the heart and arteries even in people who are otherwise healthy.

Recent finding: A University of Southern California study that looked at 735 patients for more than 12 years found that chronic stress and anxiety were better predictors of future cardiovascular events (such as a heart attack) than other risk factors. The researchers estimate that those who reduce or stabilize their stress levels are 50% to 60% less likely to have a heart attack than those who experience increasing stress.

TOXIC OVER TIME

Researchers have known for a long time that sudden traumatic events can trigger heart problems. Three years after the 9/11 terrorist attacks, for example, study participants—most of whom watched the attacks on live television—were questioned about their stress levels. Those who still were severely stressed were 53% more likely to have heart problems, and twice as likely to develop high blood pressure, as those with lower stress levels.

It appears that even "normal" stress—financial pressures or an unhappy job situation—is dangerous when it continues for a long time. It's estimated that more than 75% of visits to primary care physicians are linked to stress-related disorders.

What happens: Chronic stress increases vascular resistance, the main cause of high blood pressure. It increases the activity of platelets, cell-like structures in blood that clump together and trigger most heart attacks. It increases levels of cortisol, adrenaline and other stress hormones that promote arterial inflammation.

Doctors have been slow to acknowledge stress as a major cardiovascular risk factor. This is partly because stress (like pain) is subjective and highly individual—it's difficult to quantify, because everyone has different stress triggers and experiences stress differently. One lawyer might thrive on hectic 16-hour days, while another might react with high anxiety.

Stress can't be directly measured, but tests show its toxic effects. When laboratory subjects who are asked to count backward from 100 by eights get increasingly frustrated, there is a corresponding increase in their heart rate, adrenaline and substances linked to inflammation, such as C-reactive protein and interleukins.

STRESS REDUCTION WORKS

We can only partly control our emotional environments—stress-causing events can't always be avoided. But we can greatly change the ways in which we react to stress. People who do this can significantly lower their cardiovascular risks.

In one study, patients with heart disease were divided into three groups and followed for up to five years. Those in one group practiced stress reduction. Those in the other groups were treated either with an exercise program or with standard medical care. (The standard-care group maintained their regular medical regimen and did not participate in an exercise or stress-management program.)

Only 10% of those in the stress-control group had a subsequent heart attack or required bypass surgery or angioplasty, compared with 21% in the exercise group and 30% in the medical-care group.

BREATHE

The traditional techniques for reducing stress, such as yoga, are helpful but typically too complicated and time-consuming for most people. My colleagues and I have developed a simpler approach that anyone can do in about 15 minutes a day. It goes by the acronym B-R-E-A-T-H-E, which stands for Begin, Relax, Envision, Apply, Treat, Heal and End.

- **Begin.** Pick a time of day when you won't be interrupted for 15 minutes. Find a comfortable location. Many patients use their bedrooms, but any quiet, private place will work.
- **Relax.** This phase of the exercise is meant to elicit the relaxation response, a physiological process that reduces stress hormones and slows electrical activity in the brain. It also reduces inflammation.
- **Sit or lie quietly.** Focus so completely on your breathing that there isn't room in your mind for anything else. Inhale slowly and deeply through your nose. Then exhale just as slowly through your mouth. Each inhalation and exhalation should take about seven seconds.

Repeat the breathing cycle seven times. You'll know you're ready to go to the next step when your body is so relaxed that it feels as if all of your weight is supported by the chair or bed rather than by your muscles.

- **Envision.** Spend a few minutes imagining that every part of your heart—the arteries, muscles, valves and the electrical system—is strong and healthy. Form a mental picture (it doesn't have to be anatomically accurate) of the heart pumping blood and sending nourishment throughout your body. Hold the mental image for several minutes.

Studies using PET scans show that people who imagine that they are performing an action activate the same part of the brain that is involved when they actually do that action. Imagining a healthy heart literally can make the heart healthier.

- **Apply.** It's up to you when (and how often) you perform this relaxation exercise. Most people can find 15 minutes a day to take a mental break from stress to keep their hearts healthy. Others also use this technique when they notice that their stress levels are rising.

During a hectic day at work, for example, you might take a break for 15 minutes to calm down with conscious breathing and visualization.

- **Treat and heal.** I encourage patients to embrace the pleasurable aspects of this exercise. Don't consider it a chore. It's more like a spa treatment than a physical workout.

The healing aspect can be strongly motivating, particularly if you already have a history of heart disease. Every time you do this exercise, you are strengthening the neural networks that connect the heart and brain. This can lead to a decrease in heart arrhythmias (irregularities), an increase in immune-cell activity and even better sleep.

•**End.** Finish each relaxation session by making a mental checklist of what you have achieved. You have imagined that your heart and arteries are healthy. You have reduced stress hormones, and you are feeling more relaxed and energized than you did before.

The results are long-lasting. People who practice this for a few weeks will find themselves dealing with unexpected stressful events productively and in a calm, focused manner.

REPORT #46
Breakthrough! First New Lupus Drug in More Than 50 Years

FDA news release.
Los Angeles Times.

The US Food and Drug Administration (FDA) gave lupus patients their first new treatment option in more than 50 years when it approved Benlysta as a way to ease the painful symptoms of this debilitating autoimmune disorder.

Injected directly into a vein, Benlysta is the first drug designed to target a protein that may reduce the number of abnormal B cells believed to be at the root of lupus, the FDA said in a news release. The last lupus drugs approved by the agency were Plaquenil (*hydroxychloroquine*) and corticosteroids; both were given the agency's blessing in 1955. Back in 1948, aspirin was approved to treat the disease.

ABOUT LUPUS

Lupus strikes women far more often than men, and symptoms typically first appear between the ages of 15 and 44. The joints, skin, kidneys, lungs, heart and brain can all be affected, and when symptoms flare up they include swelling in the joints or joint pain, light sensitivity, fever, chest pain, hair loss and fatigue, the FDA said.

According to the agency, there are between 300,000 and 1.5 million lupus sufferers in the United States. Black women are three times more likely than white women to get the disorder.

NEW TREATMENT

"Benlysta, when used with existing therapies, may be an important new treatment approach for health-care professionals and patients looking to help manage symptoms associated with this disease," said Dr. Curtis Rosebraugh, director of the Office of Drug Evaluation II in the FDA's Center for Drug Evaluation and Research.

Benlysta's arrival has been much heralded because it comes on the heels of decades of disappointing efforts to craft new treatments for lupus, Sandra Raymond, president of Lupus Foundation of America, told the *Times*.

"It's an historic day. It really does open a door," Raymond told the newspaper. "Not that Benlysta is a miracle drug. It's not. I think the lupus community is sanguine about that. But they know that there are other companies coming behind" (Human Genome).

REPORT #47
Chest Pains— What They Mean… What to Do

Albert Miller, MD, professor of clinical medicine (cardiology) at Northwestern University's Feinberg School of Medicine and a clinical cardiologist at Northwestern Memorial Hospital, both in Chicago. He is author of *Chest Pain—When & When Not to Worry* (Selfhelp Success). He has authored or coauthored more than 120 medical journal articles on cardiovascular disease.

Virtually everyone feels chest pain at some point—and for good reason. Any of the organs in the chest, as well as the chest wall itself, can cause pain.

While severe pain is clearly something that you should pay close attention to, lesser degrees of pain also can indicate trouble. Surprisingly, mild chest pain can signal a heart attack, while some severe pains may not always be serious (such as pains due to sore muscles).

Your health—and, in some cases, your life—depends on knowing when chest pain indicates a serious condition that needs immediate attention.

Important: If you experience any feeling in your chest that's new or that you don't understand—especially if it persists—consult a doctor.

Some possible causes of chest pain—and what each may mean…

IT'S THE HEART!

• **Heart attack.**

Typical symptoms: Pressure, squeezing or heaviness behind the breastbone in the center of your chest, which is often associated with nausea, sweating, light-headedness or shortness of breath.

This could signal a heart attack, caused when blood flow to the heart is cut off by a blood clot in a coronary artery. Many people mistakenly think the heart is located on the left side of the chest (because they feel their heartbeat there), but it's actually just a little left of center—so pain in the mid-chest should be taken seriously.

What you may not know: It's common to have a history of milder chest pain in the center of the chest preceding (by up to two weeks in some cases) the more severe pain of a heart attack. Pain from a heart attack also can radiate to one or both shoulders and arms (especially the left) or to the neck or jaw.

If you suffer mid-chest pain, call 911 and get to a hospital emergency department as quickly as possible! Do not wait to see if the pain goes away. Prompt treatment could minimize damage to your heart muscle and may save your life.

• **Stable angina pectoris.**

Typical symptoms: A crushing pain or mild to moderate squeezing, tightness or heaviness in the middle of the chest brought on by physical exertion, emotional stress or cold weather—all of which can increase the work of the heart. Pain is relieved by rest and usually lasts five minutes or less.

The pain of angina pectoris indicates insufficient blood flow to the heart muscle, usually due to partial blockages from fatty deposits that narrow one or more coronary arteries. While this pain isn't a medical emergency like a heart attack, it's a sign that you need to schedule a doctor visit.

• **Unstable angina pectoris.**

Typical symptoms: Unexplained pain (not necessarily severe) in the middle of the chest, tightness, constriction, squeezing or heaviness…and/or pain in the neck, left shoulder or left arm. These symptoms persist and/or may occur while you're at rest or awaken you at night.

But any change of symptom pattern may also indicate unstable angina.

Associated with significantly impaired blood flow to the heart muscle, unstable angina pectoris frequently indicates an impending heart attack. If you experience these symptoms, go to a hospital emergency department immediately.

THE HEART IS NOT THE CULPRIT

• **Lung condition.**

Typical symptoms: A sharp pain in either side of the chest, made worse by breathing.

This may indicate a lung problem such as pneumonia…pleurisy (inflammation of the surface lining of a lung)…or a blood clot that formed elsewhere (usually in a leg vein), broke off and traveled to the lungs. A pulmonary blood clot is life-threatening and requires hospitalization and treatment.

• **Aortic dissection.**

Typical symptoms: Usually excruciating, tearing pain in the chest or between the shoulder blades.

This pain arises from "dissection" of the aorta (the large artery that carries blood from the left ventricle to the rest of the body) and occurs when blood from the aorta burrows between the layers of its wall. This condition is a major emergency requiring immediate medical care.

LESS SERIOUS CHEST PAINS

• **Acid reflux.**

Typical symptoms: A burning discomfort in the middle of the chest that may radiate to the throat, commonly after eating spicy food or drinking alcohol or coffee. Acid reflux (in which stomach contents wash up into the esophagus) is not an emergency but warrants treatment if it is recurrent.

• **Musculoskeletal problem.**

Typical symptoms: Pain in the chest, shoulder or upper back that is aggravated by specific movements, such as reaching for an object or putting an item on a high shelf.

These pains are typically due to a musculoskeletal problem, such as a strained muscle or tendon or arthritis. Each merits medical attention, but none is a serious health threat.

Important: Sharp, shooting pains in the chest that last just a few seconds also can be musculoskeletal in origin. These transitory pains are usually insignificant.

• **Neck problem.**

Typical symptoms: Pain on the side of the neck and/or across the right or left shoulder, and sometimes also in the upper chest on the same side of the affected shoulder.

This can be caused by a ruptured spinal disk in the neck. Treatment depends on the severity of the problem.

• **Panic attack.**

Typical symptoms: Breathing problems (such as shortness of breath or hyperventilation), perhaps accompanied by chest discomfort. These symptoms should be evaluated by a doctor.

REPORT #48
Standard Heart Tests Fail to Show True Risks

James Ehrlich, MD, clinical associate professor of endocrinology at the University of Colorado, Denver. The chief medical officer of United Cardio Systems, based in Castle Rock, Colorado.

You may think that you are at low risk for a heart attack because the heart tests that your doctor has ordered had "negative" results. The standard blood test that you received may show that your cholesterol and triglyceride levels are fine. And you may have even received a clean bill of health after taking a cardiac stress test (exercising on a treadmill while heart rhythms are electronically monitored).

Surprising fact: Those two standard heart tests miss many high-risk individuals with early heart disease. For example, a study published in the *Journal of the American College of Cardiology* found that 95% of women who had heart attacks at age 65 or younger were considered low risk.

For the greatest protection: In addition to the standard heart tests, all adults should consider receiving the highly accurate heart tests described in this article, which are not regularly ordered by most physicians but serve as stronger predictors of cardiovascular disease.

Why don't more doctors have conversations with their patients about these important tests? Many physicians closely adhere to the guidelines of the government's Preventive Services Task Force, whose evidence-based recommendations tend to include tests that are less sophisticated and less expensive.

But if your primary care physician or cardiologist does not mention these tests, ask him/her which ones might be right for you. The results will provide the best possible information for your doctor to create a customized medical and lifestyle regimen that can help prevent heart attacks and strokes.

CORONARY CALCIUM CT SCAN

This radiological imaging test—also called a CT heart scan—detects and quantifies calcified plaque, a marker for atherosclerosis (fatty buildup in the arteries). This test is up to 10 times more predictive of future heart problems than a cholesterol test and can detect early heart disease that often goes undetected by a stress test.

My advice: Men over age 35 and women over age 40 with one to two risk factors for cardiovascular disease are good candidates for screening with a heart scan. Risk factors include being overweight…having hypertension, diabetes (or prediabetes), high LDL "bad" cholesterol, low HDL "good" cholesterol, elevated triglycerides, a family history of heart disease…and/or smoking.

Risks: Cardiac CT tests expose patients to ionizing radiation (the same type used in X-rays), which has been linked to an increased risk for cancer. Heart scans, such as electron-beam CT scans and late-generation spiral CT scans, now are performed at lower radiation doses—the equivalent of 10 to 25 chest X-rays is typical. These CT scans use faster speeds than standard CT scans to produce the image, are accurate and expose you to less radiation.

Cost and coverage: $150 to $500 and may be covered by insurance.

CAROTID TEST

An ultrasound test of the carotid (neck) arteries leading to the brain does not involve radiation and measures two important conditions that help predict cardiovascular disease—the dangerous presence of plaque and the thickness of the two inner layers of each artery (the intima and media).

The carotid test is a stronger predictor of a future stroke than coronary calcium and a moderate predictor of heart attack risk.

My advice: I recommend this test for men over age 35 and women over age 40 with one to two risk factors such as hypertension and/or a family history of heart disease or stroke. People with such risk factors as high cholesterol and type 2 diabetes also may benefit from the test.

Results: If there is any noticeable plaque or the thickness of the intima/media is in the top 25% for people of your age, sex and ethnicity, you are at a higher than desirable cardiovascular risk and should pay close attention to all risk factors—especially hypertension.

Cost and coverage: $100 to $500 and often is covered by insurance.

ADVANCED LIPOPROTEIN ANALYSIS

Advanced lipoprotein analysis includes blood tests that measure hidden risk factors such as…

• **Lp(a),** a dangerous particle that often is elevated in families with a history of premature heart attacks.

• **ApoB/ApoAI,** a ratio of dangerous particles to protective particles.

My advice: This analysis is especially useful for people with heart disease that occurs in the absence of risk factors or who have a family history of premature heart disease (heart attack before age 55 in a father or brother and before age 65 in a mother or sister, for example). Those with type 2 diabetes (or prediabetes) or "metabolic syndrome"—often with a bulging waistline, hypertension, low HDL, elevated triglycerides and/or elevated blood sugar—also are good candidates.

Cost and coverage: Varies widely from as little as $40 to as much as $400—often covered by insurance.

However, not all labs perform these tests. Labs that perform advanced lipoprotein analysis: Atherotech (*www.atherotech.com*)…Berkeley Heart Lab (*www.bhlinc.com*)…Boston Heart Diagnostics (*www.bostonheartdiagnostics.com*)…Health Diagnostic Laboratory (*www.hdlabinc.com*)…LipoScience (*www.liposcience.com*)…and SpectraCell (*www.spectracell.com*).

OTHER BIOMARKERS

• **Lp-PLA2 (PLAC test).** This blood test, which measures inflammation in blood vessels themselves, is a powerful predictor of the most common type of stroke (ischemic stroke). The test is more specific for vascular disease than the commonly ordered test for C-reactive protein (which is elevated with any type of inflammation in the body).

Cost and coverage: About $50 to $200 and may be covered by insurance.

• **BNP or NT-proBNP (B-type natriuretic peptide).** This is an early indicator of a weakening heart muscle (even before overt heart failure) and an excellent test for managing patients with heart failure. The test can also be used to help predict risk for heart attack.

Cost and coverage: About $50 to $250 and may be covered by insurance.

ASPIRIN RESISTANCE TESTING

Aspirin helps stop blood components called platelets from sticking together, which reduces the risk for an artery-plugging blood clot. A daily "baby" aspirin (81 mg) or higher doses usually are prescribed for anyone who has had a heart attack or stroke…or for someone who is at risk for either condition.

However, 25% of people are aspirin resistant—the drug doesn't effectively prevent platelet "stickiness."

Aspirin resistance testing measures a urinary metabolite (11-dehydrothromboxane B2), which is high if you are aspirin resistant.

Who should be tested: Anyone taking aspirin to treat or prevent cardiovascular disease.

Cost and coverage: $30 to $150 and often covered by insurance.

Good news: Recent research published in the *Journal of the American College of Cardiology* shows that supplementing the diet with omega-3 fatty acids can overcome aspirin resistance.

SOBERING STATISTICS

About 81 million American adults have cardiovascular disease. This may include narrowed, blocked arteries (coronary artery disease)…irregular heartbeats (arrhythmia)…and/or a weakened heart muscle (heart failure).

Every year, 1.5 million of those Americans have heart attacks and 500,000 of them die. Another 800,000 have strokes, 140,000 of whom die.

REPORT #49
Up to 80% of Heart Failure Cases Could Be Prevented

Gregg Fonarow, MD, professor of medicine and director of the Ahmanson-UCLA Cardiomyopathy Center, Los Angeles. He directs the UCLA Cardiology Fellowship Training Program and is codirector of the Preventive Cardiology Program. He has published more than 400 research studies and clinical trials in heart failure management and preventive cardiology.

About five million Americans suffer from heart failure, but this disease can be avoided.

Unfortunately, few patients and doctors are aggressive enough in following through on treatment of the risk factors, such as high blood pressure (hypertension), elevated cholesterol and atherosclerosis (fatty buildup in the arteries), that can lead to heart failure.

Without adequate treatment, the heart muscle becomes damaged and weakened to the point that it can no longer adequately pump blood throughout the body.

It sounds obvious and it may be inconvenient, but research shows that about 50% to 80% of all cases of heart failure could be prevented with lifestyle modifications and/or better management of the risk factors.

AN UNDERTREATED DISEASE

Over time, the impaired circulation that marks heart failure can cause "congestion" of blood in the lower legs, lungs, liver or abdomen—often leading to fatigue, weakness and shortness of breath.

When heart failure is inadequately treated, many serious complications can result, including pump failure (when the heart malfunctions and pumps inefficiently)…sudden arrhythmias (abnormal heart rhythms)…kidney failure (due to reduced blood flow)…and heart attack or stroke (from clots triggered by impaired circulation).

There isn't a cure for heart failure. The challenge is to relieve symptoms and restore most of the heart's normal function. When heart failure is severe, pumping devices or even a heart transplant may be considered. *Latest findings on treating heart failure…*

MOST EFFECTIVE TREATMENTS

In addition to controlling the conditions that often accompany heart failure, patients can reduce heart symptoms with a combination of medications…

• **Beta-blockers.** They're among the most effective drugs for heart failure because they slow the heart rate, reduce the heart's workload and protect the heart against harmful neurohormones (chemical messengers that overproduce and cause damage in heart failure).

Patients treated with beta-blockers can experience an improvement in ejection fraction (a measure of the heart's squeezing ability) of seven to 10 percentage points, which is enough to reduce symptoms, such as fatigue. Their risk of dying from heart failure can be reduced by 30% to 40%.

Two drugs, which are often underdosed, have been shown to be effective.

For best results: Metoprolol (Lopressor) taken at a dose of 200 mg daily…or *carvedilol* (Coreg) at a dose of 25 mg twice daily.

• **Aldosterone antagonists.** These drugs, which include *spironolactone* (Aldactone), are known as potassium-sparing diuretics because they're less likely than older drugs to deplete potassium from the body. Most people with heart failure require diuretics to remove excess fluids from the body since the heart's inefficient pumping action can lead to fluid buildup.

Troubling research: Researchers at the University of California, Los Angeles, published a study showing that only about one-third of patients who should be taking these drugs are getting them. Many doctors are reluctant to prescribe aldosterone antagonists because these drugs require frequent monitoring and dose adjustments to prevent increased levels of potassium.

However, aldosterone antagonists can reverse scarring of the heart and improve its pumping ability. They improve survival by at least 30% and also reduce the risk for sudden death from heart disease.

For best results: A typical starting dose of spironolactone is 12.5 mg once daily, but your dose may vary depending on your symptoms, renal function and potassium level.

• **Angiotensin receptor blockers.** These drugs, including *losartan* (Cozaar), are designed to relax blood vessels so that it's easier for the heart to pump blood.

For best results: The standard dose for losartan used to be 50 mg, but new research indicates that 150 mg can significantly reduce the need for hospitalization due to uncontrolled heart failure symptoms. Side effects include cough, elevated potassium, dizziness and headache.

WHEN MORE HELP IS NEEDED

If you have made lifestyle changes (such as reducing fat in your diet and getting regular exercise) and have received maximum treatment with medication but still suffer symptoms of heart failure, you may need even more help.

• **Cardiac resynchronization is a relatively new treatment in which electrodes are placed on the left and right sides of the heart.** Electrical impulses delivered to the electrodes from an implanted biventrical pacemaker paces both sides of the lower chambers of the heart, improving the heart's pumping action. A battery pack that is a little smaller than a deck of cards is implanted under the collarbone.

How it helps: Cardiac resynchronization, combined with medication, can reduce hospitalizations from heart failure complications by 50%…and reduce the risk of dying from heart failure by 35% to 40%.

• **Left ventricular assist device (LVAD).** Former vice president Dick Cheney had surgery for implantation of an LVAD. This device gives a boost to the heart's main pumping chamber and helps it deliver blood to the rest of the body. The LVAD, which is surgically attached to the left ventricle and connected to a power source (such as batteries) outside the body, is an important breakthrough because the majority of patients who receive the implant may survive long enough to get a heart transplant.

One device, the HeartMate II, was approved by the FDA in April 2008. Research found that patients given this device had one-year survival rates of 68% compared with 55% with earlier-generation LVADs.

ADDITIONAL USEFUL THERAPIES

Other therapies that can help ease heart failure symptoms…

• **Omega-3 fatty acids.** In a study of nearly 7,000 heart failure patients who received either placebos or 1,000 mg of omega-3s daily, those taking omega-3s were about 10% less likely to die.

• **Intravenous iron.** Heart failure patients who are deficient in iron may improve slightly when they receive iron intravenously. This treatment isn't approved by the FDA for this use, and it hasn't been proven to prolong survival times. However, in those who are iron-deficient (even if they don't have anemia), intravenous iron may help ease symptoms. If you have heart failure, ask your doctor about having your iron levels tested.

• **Sodium and fluid restriction.** Since a high-sodium diet can significantly increase blood pressure in many people, individuals with heart failure should limit their sodium intake. The optimal sodium intake for heart failure patients hasn't been established, but they are usually advised not to exceed 1,500 mg daily.

Fluid restriction is also important, particularly for those who have congestion. Patients who struggle with fluid retention should limit the amount they drink to about two liters (about 68 ounces) daily.

Caution: Heart failure patients should never take aspirin or any other nonsteroidal anti-inflammatory drug (NSAID) without consulting a doctor. These drugs have been associated with a worsening of heart failure symptoms. *Acetaminophen* (Tylenol) may be a better option. Certain diabetes drugs, such as *rosiglitazone* (Avandia) and *pioglitazone* (Actos), also should be avoided by people with heart failure.

REPORT #50
Say Good-Bye to Your Diabetes Medication

Mark A. Stengler, NMD, naturopathic medical doctor and leading authority on the practice of alternative and integrated medicine. Dr. Stengler is author of the *Health Revelations* newsletter, author of *The Natural Physician's Healing Therapies* (Bottom Line Books), founder and medical director of the Stengler Center for Integrative Medicine in Encinitas, California, and adjunct associate clinical professor at the National College of Natural Medicine in Portland, Oregon. *http://markstengler.com*

Some of my patients who have type 2 diabetes are able to keep the disease under control with diet and exercise. Lucky them! But for other diabetes patients, that's not enough and they must take pharmaceutical medications.

There is another natural treatment option for diabetes patients who currently take pharmaceutical medications. Research has found that a plant extract called *berberine* can control diabetes as well as, or better than, common medications such as *metformin* (Glucophage) and *rosiglitazone* (Avandia). And it does this with no side effects—and without damaging the liver, as some medications do. *Here's how berberine can help people with diabetes…*

A naturally occurring chemical compound, berberine is found in the roots and stems of several plants, including *Hydrastis canadensis* (goldenseal), *Coptis chinensis* (coptis or goldthread) and *Berberis aquifolium* (Oregon grape). Long used as a remedy in Chinese and Ayurvedic medicines, berberine is known for its antimicrobial properties and as a treatment for bacterial and fungal infections. Several decades ago, berberine was used to treat diarrhea in patients in China. That was when doctors noticed that the blood sugar levels of diabetes patients were lower after taking the herbal extract—and berberine began to be investigated for this purpose.

Over the past 20 years, there has been much research on berberine and its effectiveness in treating diabetes. In 2008, Chinese researchers published a study in *Metabolism* in which adults with newly diagnosed type 2 diabetes were given 500 milligrams (mg) of either berberine or the drug metformin three times a day for three months. Researchers found that berberine did as good a job as metformin at regulating glucose metabolism, as indicated by hemoglobin A1C (a measure of blood glucose over several weeks)...fasting blood glucose...blood sugar after eating...and level of insulin after eating. Berberine even reduced the amount of insulin needed to turn glucose into energy by 45%! In addition, those taking berberine had noticeably lower trigylceride and total cholesterol levels than those taking metformin.

In a recent study in *Metabolism*, Chinese researchers compared people with type 2 diabetes who took either 1,000 mg daily of berberine or daily doses of metformin or rosiglitazone. After two months, berberine had lowered subjects' fasting blood glucose levels by an average of about 30%, an improvement over the rosiglitazone group and almost as much as people in the metformin group. Berberine also reduced subjects' hemoglobin A1C by 18%—equal to rosiglitazone and, again, almost as good as metformin. In addition, berberine lowered serum insulin levels by 28.2% (indicating increased insulin sensitivity)...lowered triglycerides by 17.5%...and actually improved liver enzyme levels. Pharmaceutical medications, on the other hand, have the potential to harm the liver.

These were remarkable findings. Here was a botanical that was holding up to scientific scrutiny—and performing as well as, or better than, some drugs that patients had been taking for diabetes for years.

HOW BERBERINE WORKS IN THE BODY

Berberine helps to lower blood glucose in several ways. One of its primary mechanisms involves stimulating the activity of the genes responsible for manufacturing and activating insulin receptors, which are critical for controlling blood glucose.

Berberine also has an effect on blood sugar regulation through activation of *incretins*, gastrointestinal hormones that affect the amount of insulin released by the body after eating.

HOW BERBERINE CAN HELP

I recommend berberine to my patients with newly diagnosed type 2 diabetes to reduce their blood sugar and prevent them from needing pharmaceutical drugs. When a diet, exercise and supplement program (including supplements such as chromium) is already helping a diabetes patient, I don't recommend that he/she switch to berberine.

Some patients are able to take berberine—and make dietary changes—and stop taking diabetes drugs altogether. People with severe diabetes can use berberine in conjunction with medication—and this combination treatment allows for fewer side effects and better blood sugar control. I don't recommend berberine for prediabetes unless diet and exercise are not effective. Berberine is sold in health-food stores and online in tablet and capsule form. The dosage I typically recommend for all diabetes patients is 500 mg twice daily.

For patients with diabetes who want to use berberine, I recommend talking to your doctor about taking this supplement. It's also important for every patient with diabetes to participate in a comprehensive diet and exercise program.

Note that berberine helps patients with type 2 diabetes, not type 1 diabetes (in which the body does not produce enough insulin).

REPORT #51
The "Cooking Oil Cure" For High Blood Pressure

Inter-American Society of Hypertension scientific meeting, San Antonio, Texas.
American Heart Association news release

Using sesame oil instead of other cooking oils helps reduce high blood pressure and lower the amount of medication required to control high blood pressure, according to a study by researchers in India.

The study looked at the effect of sesame oil on 328 people with hypertension who were taking 10 to 30 milligrams (mg) a day of the calcium channel blocker *nifedipine*, which lowers blood pressure by relaxing muscles in the walls of arteries.

The average age of those studied was 58 years. They had moderate to severe long-term hypertension but no history of stroke or heart disease.

They consumed an average of 35 grams of sesame oil a day for 60 days. Their blood pressure was measured at the start of the study, every 15 days during the study and on day 60.

The study found that by using sesame oil as their sole cooking oil, participants lowered their blood pressure readings from an average 166/101 to 134/84.6.

Also, the average dose of nifedipine taken by the participants was reduced from 22.7 mg per day to 7.45 mg per day by the end of the study.

WHAT DO THE BLOOD PRESSURE NUMBERS MEAN?

The American Heart Association (*www.heart.org*) says that in blood pressure readings, the top (systolic) number represents the pressure while the heart is beating and the bottom (diastolic) number represents the pressure when the heart is resting between beats. The association says optimal blood pressure is 115/75 or lower.

REPORT #52
How Brain Scientist Jill Bolte Taylor Came Back From a Stroke

Jill Bolte Taylor, PhD, a neuroanatomist affiliated with the Indiana University School of Medicine in Indianapolis. She is a national spokesperson for the Harvard Brain Tissue Resource Center, which collects human brain tissue for research. The author of *My Stroke of Insight: A Brain Scientist's Personal Journey* (Plume), she was named one of *Time* magazine's 100 Most Influential People in the World for 2008.

In 1996, Jill Bolte Taylor, PhD, a 37-year-old brain scientist, had a severe hemorrhagic (bleeding) stroke in the left hemisphere of her brain.

Taylor's cognitive abilities degenerated rapidly in the hours following the stroke. Bleeding affected the motor cortex (paralyzing her right arm)…the sensory cortex (making it difficult for her to see or hear)…and the brain's language centers (making it difficult for her to speak).

After struggling to call for help, she was taken to the hospital, where she underwent surgery two-and-a-half weeks later to remove a golf ball–sized blood clot in her brain.

Today, Taylor is completely recovered—all of her physical, cognitive and emotional abilities are intact. Her eight-year recovery refutes the widely held belief that if a stroke survivor doesn't regain a particular ability within six months, it will never be regained.

Taylor, a neuroanatomist (a scientist specializing in the anatomy of the brain) now lectures widely about her stroke recovery. The strategies she shares can be used by all those who have had a debilitating ischemic stroke (in which a blood clot stops blood supply to an area of the brain) or any severe brain injury…

STEP 1: MOVE TO RECOVER

People who survive a stroke often experience crushing fatigue due to the damage that occurs to brain cells (neurons)—this affects their energy levels and abilities to process information. Simple tasks, such as changing the position of your body or even opening your eyes, are extraordinarily difficult. But the same activities that restore physical strength also force individual neurons to reconnect and communicate with one another—a process that is essential for post-stroke neurological recovery.

Helpful: Any physical activity is beneficial—even basic movements, such as standing up or sitting down.

Important: When you feel rested and capable of expending the necessary energy, you should push yourself to do more and more physically each day. As I gained strength, I progressed to trying more difficult activities, such as standing at the sink and doing dishes.

STEP 2: ESCAPE THE MENTAL NOISE

Neurons that are damaged by a stroke are unable to process normal stimuli, such as bright lights or the sound of a television. As a result, visual or auditory distractions may be interpreted by the brain as mental "noise." Saturating the brain with such stimuli may make it much harder for the neurons to recover and may impede the retention of new information.

Helpful: After any kind of stroke or other brain trauma, alternate periods of sleep with briefer periods (about 20 minutes) of learning and cognitive challenges (such as those described below). Periods of sleep (as much as needed until waking up naturally) allow the brain to assimilate information that is gleaned during periods of wakefulness.

STEP 3: WORK THE MIND

The brain has remarkable "plasticity" (the ability to form new connections between the surviving neurons). After a stroke, if there is damage to the brain areas that control movement, sensory perceptions and cognition, you need to challenge these areas.

Examples...

- **Multiple-choice questions.** My mother, who was my primary caregiver, understood that asking "yes" or "no" questions didn't force me to think hard enough. That's why she asked me open-ended questions—for example, did I want minestrone soup or a grilled cheese sandwich? Each question forced me to relearn words.

- **Simple puzzles.** If you've had a serious stroke, putting together a simple jigsaw puzzle may be a huge challenge. You might not recognize shapes or colors. You might not have the dexterity to put the pieces together. But doing such a puzzle is a superb exercise because it forces you to work different parts of the brain at the same time.

- **Reading.** It's among the hardest tasks because, for many stroke patients, the entire concept of letters and words is lost—temporarily for some stroke survivors, but permanently for others. I had to relearn everything from scratch—that the squiggles that make up letters have names...that combinations of letters make sounds...and that combinations of sounds make words.

Helpful: I started with children's picture books, which would be appropriate for most stroke patients who are relearning to read.

STEP 4: THE SIMPLEST STEPS

Healthy people can't begin to comprehend how complicated things seem after a stroke. When I first started walking, for example, I didn't understand the concept of sidewalk cracks. Each time I saw one, I had to stop and analyze whether it was important.

Helpful: Caregivers need to break down tasks to the simplest levels. For example, a stroke patient might not understand how to sit up in bed. He/she might need to spend days just learning how to shift body weight. In my case, I had to learn to simply hold an eating utensil before I could imagine raising it to my mouth.

STEP 5: FOCUS ON ABILITIES

When you've had a stroke, the extent of your disabilities can be overwhelming. It took me eight years before I was fully recovered. Patients can easily get frustrated and quit trying. At that point, if a patient is not aware of what recovery step needs to be taken next, he may never actually take that next step. It's normal for a stroke survivor to reach a recovery plateau, to continue to learn, then hit another plateau. There are many plateaus along the way.

Helpful: Even if progress seems exceptionally slow, remind a person who has had a stroke of the smallest successes—it may be something as simple as once again being able to hold a fork securely.

If you are the stroke survivor, use small triumphs as inspiration. In my case, it was embarrassing to drool in front of strangers, but I would remind myself that I had at least managed to swallow.

After my stroke, I never imagined that I would regain enough of my abilities to return to a career as a scientist and teacher. I've managed to do both—in fact, at the same level and intensity. My stroke recovery gave me an opportunity to start my life again.

REPORT #53
Can Diet Soda Boost Your Stroke Risk?

Hannah Gardener, ScD, epidemiologist, University of Miami Miller School of Medicine.
Patrick Lyden, MD, chief, neurology, Cedars-Sinai Medical Center, Los Angeles.
International Stroke Conference, Los Angeles.

Diet soda fans who drink the beverages every day may be cutting down on calories, but they also might be boosting their risk of stroke, recent research suggests.

"In our study, we saw a significant increased risk among those who drank diet soda daily and not regular soda," said Hannah Gardener, ScD, an epidemiologist at the University of Miami Miller School of Medicine, who presented her research at the International Stroke Conference in Los Angeles.

Why the link? "It's unknown at this point," she said.

BACKGROUND

Stroke is the third leading cause of death, behind heart disease and cancer, in the United States. More than 137,000 people a year die from stroke, according to the American Stroke Association.

Previous research has found that those who drank more than one soft drink a day, whether regular or diet, were more likely than nondrinkers to have metabolic syndrome, a cluster of risk factors including high blood pressure, elevated triglycerides (blood fats), low levels of good cholesterol, high fasting blood sugar and large waists. Metabolic syndrome, in turn, raises the risk of diabetes and cardiovascular disease, experts agree.

THE STUDY

Dr. Gardener and her colleagues evaluated the soda habits of 2,564 people enrolled in the large Northern Manhattan Study (NOMAS) to see if there was an association, if any, with stroke. The participants were 69 years of age, on average, and completed food questionnaires about the type of soda they drank and how often.

During the average nine-year follow-up, 559 vascular events occurred, including strokes caused by hemorrhage and those caused by clots, known as ischemic strokes.

The researchers controlled for such factors as age, gender, ethnicity, physical activity, calorie intake, smoking and alcohol drinking habits and still found that those who drank diet soda daily—compared with those who drank no soda—were 61% more likely to have a vascular event.

The researchers then controlled for the presence of metabolic syndrome, vascular disease in the limbs and heart disease history. The link still held, but at a lower 48%.

IMPLICATION

While the study found a possible association between diet soda and stroke risk, it did not demonstrate a cause and effect. And experts note that research presented at meetings has not been subjected to the same type of rigorous scrutiny given to research published in peer-reviewed medical journals.

"If our study is replicated," Dr. Gardener said, "it would suggest diet soda is not optimal."

EXPERT COMMENTARY

Patrick Lyden, MD, chief of neurology at Cedars-Sinai Medical Center in Los Angeles, reviewed the findings but was not involved in the research. "My first thought was that the correlation was accidental," he said.

But he said the science in the study looks sound. "There still could be some sort of accidental correlation," he said. What to do? "Wait for repeated studies to show a risk and in the meantime, all things in moderation."

He tells his patients to avoid soda, whether diet or regular, on a daily basis. "An occasional soda never hurt anybody," he said. "Once or twice a week to me seems to be rational."

REPORT #54
How to Lose 12 Pounds…in Just 17 Days

Mike Moreno, MD, physician in charge of primary care and coordinator for new physician education at Kaiser Permanente in San Diego. Dr. Moreno is the author of *The 17 Day Diet* (Free Press).

According to conventional wisdom, anyone who loses weight rapidly (more than a pound or two a week) will invariably regain the lost pounds because the diet will be too strict to maintain. But some researchers are now finding evidence that slow isn't necessarily better when it comes to weight loss.

Recent research: A study in the *International Journal of Behavioral Medicine* analyzed data from 262 middle-aged obese women.

Result: The fast weight losers dropped more pounds overall and maintained their weight loss longer than the gradual weight losers.

Good news: With rapid weight loss, most people can boost their metabolism, combat fat storage and help prevent obesity-related diseases, such as diabetes and certain types of cancer—all without feeling deprived of satisfying food.

Sound impossible? I've seen thousands of people lose weight by following what I call the 17 Day Diet.*

Why 17 days? This is roughly the amount of time it takes for your body's metabolism to adapt to a change in calories. By varying your diet at 17-day intervals, you "trick" your metabolism into functioning at its maximum efficiency to help you reach your target weight.

Four simple cycles to follow…

Cycle 1: **Cleanse Your System.** For the first 17 days, the goal is to "cleanse" your system by eating lots of lean protein, such as poultry and fish. Lean protein requires more energy to digest than carbohydrates, so it burns additional calories and helps control your blood sugar. Protein also fights food cravings.

During this cycle, you're also allowed as many vegetables as you like. You will need to temporarily cut out all grains, potatoes, pasta and desserts. Doing this helps you avoid the dramatic fluctuations in blood sugar that fuel binge eating.

Note: Use olive oil for cooking during this cycle.

Fruit is allowed but only before 2 pm—when sugar (including natural sugar from fruit) is less likely to be stored as fat.

Good fruit choices: Apples, berries, oranges, pears, plums and red grapes. These fruits are relatively low in sugar and high in fiber, which slows digestion and helps you feel full. Avoid bananas and pineapple—both contain too much natural sugar.

During this 17-day cycle, people lose an average of 10 to 12 pounds (depending on their starting weights) while eating three to four meals daily plus snacks (for a total of 1,300 calories per day for men and women). Some of this weight loss will be due to water loss—but this is also beneficial because fluid retention can contribute to fatigue.

Sample day's meals: Breakfast—two scrambled egg whites…one-half grapefruit or other fresh fruit…one cup green tea. Lunch—fish, poultry or eggs…vegetables…one cup green tea. Dinner—fish or chicken…vegetables…one cup green tea. Snack—raw, cut-up veggies.

Cycle 2: **Reset Your Metabolism.** During the second 17-day cycle, the goal is to reset the metabolism by alternating higher calorie intake (1,500 to 1,700) on even days with lower calorie intake (1,300) on odd days. Switching back and forth stimulates fat burning because it prevents your body from adapting to a certain level of daily calories.

Slow-digesting complex carbs, such as oatmeal, sweet potatoes and brown rice, are reintroduced during this cycle.

Cycle 3: **Good Eating Habits.** By now, a little more than a month since you started, your body has undergone a significant metabolic shift that will allow you to reintroduce moderate portions—and no more than two to three servings per day before 2 pm—of carbohydrates such as whole-grain breads and pastas.

If you've reached your target weight, you may proceed to cycle 4, the maintenance cycle. If not, be sure to focus on portion control

---
*Be sure to check with your doctor before you start this or any weight-loss program.

and continue to emphasize lean protein and nonstarchy vegetables, limiting carbohydrates after 2 pm until you reach cycle 4.

Cycle 4: **Weight Maintenance.** During this cycle, which is followed indefinitely to maintain your weight loss, you are more strict with yourself throughout the workweek but relax your eating habits on the weekends. From 6 pm Friday to 6 pm Sunday, you can enjoy your favorite indulgences, such as pizza or hamburgers, as long as you maintain portion control and enjoy no more than three indulgences over a single weekend. This approach allows you to eat some favorite foods in moderation while also giving your metabolism the variety it needs to function efficiently.

Rule of thumb: Weigh yourself on weekends. If you gain five pounds or more over a week's time, return to any of the earlier cycles.

OTHER SECRETS TO WEIGHT LOSS

In addition to following the cycles described earlier...

•**Get more probiotics.** New research suggests that people who have an overabundance of "bad" bacteria in the intestinal tract are more susceptible to weight gain. But healthful bacteria, known as probiotics (found in such foods as certain yogurts, sauerkraut and miso soup), control the proliferation of bad bacteria and help fight infection—and ensure that your metabolism functions effectively.

My advice: Aim to consume two daily servings of foods containing probiotics. *Examples of one probiotic serving*: Six ounces of fat-free plain yogurt or one-half cup of Breakstone LiveActive cottage cheese (which includes added probiotics).

Or: Take probiotic supplements, following label instructions.

•**Don't forget to exercise.** To avoid getting run down while you're scaling back on calories (especially the first few days of cycle 1), do only 15 to 20 minutes of walking a day.

Thereafter, aim for at least 30 minutes of aerobic exercise five days a week. Walking is a good choice, as is jogging, swimming or using a stationary bicycle or an elliptical machine. For strength training, make the exercises as aerobic as possible using lighter weights and more repetitions.

REPORT #55
Are You Taking A Drug That Isn't FDA Approved For Your Illness?

G. Caleb Alexander, MD, MS, assistant professor, department of medicine, University of Chicago, Chicago, and adjunct research associate, department of pharmacy practice, University of Illinois at Chicago School of Pharmacy.

Are the drugs your doctor is prescribing safe and effective? Who knows? In a recent survey by researchers at the University of Virginia, the University of Chicago and the University of Illinois at Chicago, almost half of physicians who responded mistakenly believed that at least one use of a drug listed in the survey was FDA-approved, when in fact, it was not. So-called off-label prescribing is both legal and common—but this survey's findings may mean that doctors are prescribing drugs when there is insufficient evidence of their efficacy and safety for a specific purpose.

CONFUSION IS COMMON

University of Chicago lead researcher G. Caleb Alexander, MD, MS, and his colleagues conducted a national random-sample survey of doctors. A total of 1,199 physicians (599 primary care doctors and 600 psychiatrists) were sent questionnaires and nearly half responded. They were asked about 22 drug-indication pairs (i.e., particular drugs prescribed for particular conditions)...and correctly identified the FDA-approved indications of just over half the drug-indication pairs. They misidentified the FDA-approval status of the rest of the drug uses examined—and that may lead them to prescribing that puts patients at serious risk. *For example...*

•**Nearly one in five thought *quetiapine* (Seroquel) was FDA-approved for dementia**

and agitation, when in fact the drug carries a strong "black box" warning that it is dangerous for elderly people with dementia.

• **One in three who prescribed *lorazepam* (Ativan) for chronic anxiety incorrectly believed that it was FDA-approved for this purpose**—in truth, the FDA advises against using it for anxiety, because it is a strong drug with a high risk of addiction.

Dr. Alexander said that there are many reasons why doctors may not be fully aware of the FDA-label status. "The amount of information that physicians must master is vast, the evidence base is constantly changing, and some would argue that physicians should focus on the evidence and not the FDA label," he noted. "In addition, some of the drug uses that we examined may have been ones that were actually promoted by the pharmaceutical industry, which leads to confusion on the part of physicians regarding the FDA-approval status."

This is dangerous territory. "The results indicate an urgent need for more effective ways to inform physicians about the level of evidence supporting off-label drug use—especially for common off-label uses that are ineffective or carry unacceptable risks of harm," warns Dr. Alexander. These findings were published in *Pharmacoepidemiology and Drug Safety*.

REVIEW YOUR MEDICATIONS

Off-label prescribing can allow physicians to anticipate valuable new drug uses before formal FDA approval and also can offer an alternative to patients who do not respond to standard treatments. At the bare minimum, however, doctors should know whether they are writing a prescription for an approved condition or an off-label use—in the latter case, it would be best if the prescription were then subject to added scrutiny before it was written. Physicians should carefully consider the safety and effectiveness off label, especially as compared with approved medications.

What steps can consumers take to make sure that doctors prescribe the most appropriate medications, whether approved or off-label? Dr. Alexander advises always asking questions about drugs your doctor prescribes—their FDA-approval status, the scientific evidence to support their use, risks and benefits, side effects, potential drug and food interactions, dosage, cost, etc. Since there may not be time to discuss every drug at each visit, Dr. Alexander notes that these questions are most important for treatments that are new on the market. It's also a good idea to do your own research to ensure that you are as educated and empowered as possible.

REPORT #56
Prozac Speeds Stroke Recovery

Francois Chollet, MD, PhD, University Hospital of Toulouse and INSERM, Toulouse, France.

Stroke patients given the antidepressant *fluoxetine* (best known by the brand name of Prozac) appear to regain more muscle function than other recovering stroke sufferers, French researchers have found.

Not surprisingly, patients on the generic Prozac were also less susceptible to depression after their stroke, the study found.

Lead researcher Francois Chollet, MD, PhD, said the study "opens a new pathway" in the treatment of the leading form of stroke, ischemic stroke, in which a blockage in a blood vessel is the cause of the attack. Dr. Chollet, from the University Hospital of Toulouse and INSERM, noted that Prozac also appears to target neurons themselves rather than trying to reopen arteries, as many other stroke medications do.

The report is published in *The Lancet Neurology*.

BACKGROUND

Paralysis and/or weakness on one side of the body are the most common disabilities after stroke. Earlier trials have suggested that antidepressants might help improve motor recovery after stroke, probably by increasing the level of serotonin in the central nervous system, the researchers explained.

Stroke is a major cause of death and long-term disability for Americans, so any agent that helps boost functionality is of great benefit.

THE STUDY

Dr. Chollet's team randomly assigned 118 ischemic stroke patients left with paralysis or weakness on one side of the body to either 20 milligrams of generic Prozac or placebo per day starting five to 10 days after their stroke.

After three months of follow-up, patients taking generic Prozac had improved their score on a measure of motor function by 34 points over their initial test, compared with a 24.3-point improvement among those receiving placebo, the researchers found.

Moreover, this statistically significant improvement was seen in arm and leg function, Dr. Chollet's group said.

The improvement meant that more patients in the generic Prozac group were able to live independently than patients in the placebo group, the researchers noted.

The drug—from the same class of selective serotonin reuptake inhibitors (SSRIs) that includes Celexa, Paxil and Zoloft—was generally well tolerated and side effects were mild. However, nausea, diarrhea and abdominal pain were more common among patients taking the antidepressant, and two of those patients suffered serious adverse events.

The generic form of Prozac is relatively cheap now, at about 30 cents per pill.

And there was an added bonus: Patients taking generic Prozac were less likely to be depressed, which suggests that giving the antidepressant after a stroke could prevent depression, the researchers say.

But Dr. Chollet noted that remaining questions persist. "How long should be the treatment period? What is the long-term effect? Can other neurological functions, such as language and vision, be improved in a similar way? Can we observe a similar action in [the rarer form of] hemorrhagic strokes? These question will have to be addressed in a short while," he said. Hemorrhagic stroke is caused by bleeding in the brain.

EXPERT REACTION

Robert G. Robinson, MD, professor and head of the department of psychiatry at the University of Iowa and coauthor of an accompanying journal editorial, said, "the implications of the study are very positive."

Dr. Robinson noted that a study that he participated in found similar results. He believes that antidepressants may aid in producing new nerve cells in the brain and also help in creating new connections between these cells.

In addition, antidepressants may also help in preventing the inflammation seen in stroke, he said.

"This study raises the question, should all patients who have a stroke be given antidepressant medication?" Dr. Robinson said. "Given the large number of people who have stroke each year, you are talking about a huge paradigm shift in the care of stroke patients. But this finding clearly raises that question."

To find the answer, "a large definitive trial" needs to be done that compares the use of antidepressants and placebo in many patients, Dr. Robinson said. He also noted that the trial should investigate whether the effects of the treatment persist over time.

But another expert suggested that generic Prozac's role in lowering post-stroke depression might account for the improvement in physical function simply by promoting more effective participation in physical therapy.

Larry B. Goldstein, MD, director of the Duke University Stroke Center, noted that that the study failed to control for the intensity or type of physical therapy that patients received after the stroke.

Those who received the antidepressant tended to be less depressed and thus might have more effectively participated in physical therapy, he reasoned.

"Because other studies show that more intensive physical therapy is associated with better recovery, it is possible that the antidepressant effect, rather than an effect on the recovery process itself, might explain the difference," Dr. Goldstein said.

REPORT #57
Pulverize Precancerous Prostate Cells

Mark A. Stengler, NMD, naturopathic medical doctor and leading authority on the practice of alternative and integrated medicine. Dr. Stengler is author of the *Health Revelations* newsletter, author of *The Natural Physician's Healing Therapies* (Bottom Line Books), founder and medical director of the Stengler Center for Integrative Medicine in Encinitas, California, and adjunct associate clinical professor at the National College of Natural Medicine in Portland, Oregon. *http://markstengler.com*

Over the course of a lifetime, one man in six eventually will be diagnosed with prostate cancer...one in 35 will die from it. Despite how common the disease is, the treatment path for prostate cancer is seldom clear. Even conventional doctors who specialize in prostate cancer frequently disagree about the best course of action.

Surgery to remove the prostate gland and perhaps the nearby lymph nodes often is recommended, yet it can have onerous side effects —including incontinence that lasts for months or years and lifelong erectile dysfunction. What's more, statistics show that surgery does not necessarily increase a man's life span.

For these reasons, many doctors now recommend a "watch and wait" approach rather than surgery. Prostate cancer usually is slow-growing, and more than 70% of the men who develop it are over age 65. The older a man is, the more likely he is to die of some other condition before his prostate cancer becomes a real threat. The American Cancer Society (*www.cancer.org*) states, "At this time, watchful waiting is a reasonable option for some men with slow-growing cancers because it is not known whether active treatment, such as surgery, radiation therapy and hormone therapy, prolongs survival."

The holistic view: For prostate cancer patients age 65 and older, as well as for some younger men whose cancer does not appear to be fast-growing, I support the decision to watch and wait before pursuing aggressive conventional treatment—with one important caveat. Instead of waiting passively while doing nothing, I recommend a proactive approach using natural therapies that may slow or halt cancer growth or even cause the cancer to diminish.

Unless noted otherwise, all supplements described below are available at health-food stores, are generally safe to take indefinitely and cause no known serious side effects.

Important: It is vital that men who have prostate cancer be monitored by an oncologist. Show your doctor this article, and discuss these natural therapies.

CUTTING-EDGE PROSTATE CARE

Aaron E. Katz, MD, associate professor of clinical urology and director of the Center of Holistic Urology at Columbia University Medical Center in New York City headed up the research on two supplements that show promise in the fight against prostate cancer. *Here is what we know so far...*

• **Zyflamend.** This unique formula from New Chapter (800-543-7279, *www.newchapter.com*) combines phytochemicals (beneficial plant chemicals) with herbal extracts from turmeric, ginger, green tea, rosemary, hu zhang (Japanese knotweed), Chinese goldthread, barberry, oregano, baikal skullcap and holy basil.

Dr. Katz's laboratory study found that Zyflamend reduced prostate cancer cell proliferation by up to 78% and may even have killed some existing prostate cancer cells.

Dr. Katz's team analyzed results of a clinical trial of Zyflamend among men at high risk for prostate cancer. The trial included 23 men, ages 46 to 75, who were diagnosed via biopsy with a type of precancerous cell proliferation called high-grade *prostatic intraepithelial neoplasia* (PIN)—a marker suggesting an 80% chance that cancer will develop within 10 years. The men also had elevated levels of prostate-specific antigen (PSA)—a substance produced by prostate gland cells and often elevated when cancer exists. Participants took one Zyflamend pill three times a day for 18 months. *Blood tests and biopsies then showed...*

• **The PIN disappeared in 62% of patients.**

• **Half of the men had decreases in PSA levels**—some by more than 50%—indicating a return to more normal prostate cell activity.

• **For all of the nine patients who did develop cancer,** the disease was the slow-growing type and confined to a small area.

If you are at risk: Based on the evidence that Zyflamend can reverse PIN and reduce PSA, I recommend taking three Zyflamend capsules daily (with meals to avoid gastric upset), continuing indefinitely, if you have any of the following…

• **An enlarged prostate** (as detected during a doctor's exam).

• **Any abnormal prostate PIN.**

• **PSA that is elevated for your age.** PSA is considered elevated if it is at or above 2.5 nanograms per milliliter (ng/ml) in your 40s… 3.5 ng/ml in your 50s…4.5 ng/ml in your 60s… or 6.5 ng/ml in your 70s.

• **An ultrasound or other imaging test showing prostate lesions.**

• **One or more immediate family members with a history of prostate cancer, if you are over age 50.**

If you have high-grade PIN or prostate cancer: In addition to taking Zyflamend, consider taking a second supplement, Prostabel, described below…

• **Prostabel.** Available online from Natural Source International (888-308-7066, *www.natural-source.com*).

Dr. Katz's team at Columbia also conducted a clinical trial on Prostabel. The study included 25 men, ages 40 to 75, with negative biopsy reports but elevated PSA levels. Participants were assigned to take from two to eight capsules of Prostabel daily for 12 months.

Preliminary findings: Prostabel significantly lowered PSA in five of the eight men. While four of the men developed cancer, their cancers were small and slow growing. Researchers were waiting to see if Prostabel suppresses cancer cell growth in the remaining 17 participants. Just one patient, who was on the highest dosage, developed liver enzyme problems as a side effect.

Surprising: Patients experienced significant improvements in urination problems common among older men, such as frequent need to urinate and slowed stream.

Recommended dosage: Three Prostabel capsules daily. Take on an empty stomach to maximize absorption—if it causes digestive upset, take with meals instead.

MORE CANCER FIGHTERS

In addition to taking Zyflamend and/or Prostabel, I recommend that men who have had a diagnosis of prostate cancer take all of the following, continuing indefinitely…

• **Zinc.** 50 milligrams (mg) daily.

Caution: Check with your doctor before taking zinc if you are undergoing chemotherapy —zinc may not be compatible with some chemotherapy drugs.

• **Copper.** Long-term zinc supplementation can lead to a copper deficiency, so also take 2 mg of copper daily.

• **Selenium.** 200 micrograms (mcg) daily.

Note: Although evidence is not conclusive, selenium has been linked to increased risk for diabetes—so have your blood sugar monitored regularly.

• **Vitamin E.** 200 international units (IU) daily of "mixed" vitamin E (as indicated on the label).

• **Calcium limit.** No more than 500 mg of supplemental calcium daily. Some evidence links high doses to increased prostate cancer risk.

Men who have been diagnosed with prostate cancer and who want a more aggressive approach can add the following and continue taking them indefinitely…

• **Indole 3-carbinol.** 400 mg daily.

• **Maitake mushroom extract.** This enhances immune function. Use capsules or tincture labeled "standardized MD-fraction."

Take 1 mg per day for every 2.2 pounds of body weight (for instance, a 165-pound man would take 75 mg daily…a 200-pound man would take 90 mg daily). Take in two divided doses on an empty stomach.

• **Beta-glucan.** 500 mg twice daily.

REPORT #58
Major Breakthrough in Brain Health

Mark A. Stengler, NMD, naturopathic medical doctor and leading authority on the practice of alternative and integrated medicine. Dr. Stengler is author of the *Health Revelations* newsletter, author of *The Natural Physician's Healing Therapies* (Bottom Line Books), founder and medical director of the Stengler Center for Integrative Medicine in Encinitas, California, and adjunct associate clinical professor at the National College of Natural Medicine in Portland, Oregon. *http://markstengler.com*

Sometimes there is such an amazing breakthrough in research that I can't wait to share it with you. This is one of those times. In a relatively new area of science known as epigenetics (which is, at its most basic, the study of changes in gene activity), researchers have found that a protein in the body known as Nrf2 has the power to turn on genes that produce a vast array of antioxidants throughout the body and particularly in the brain. These antioxidants protect our cells from damage caused by free radicals, which are known to cause disease.

Brain cells, in particular, need this protection. The brain is especially vulnerable to damage from free radicals because it uses more energy than other parts of the body and there are more damaging particles there. Free radical damage, including the resulting oxidative stress and inflammation, has been found to underlie general brain aging and many degenerative conditions of the brain, including Alzheimer's, Parkinson's, amyotrophic lateral sclerosis (ALS, or Lou Gehrig's disease) and multiple sclerosis.

One of the main Nrf2 researchers is David Perlmutter, MD, a highly regarded integrative neurologist and coauthor of several books, including *Power Up Your Brain: The Neuroscience of Enlightenment* (Hay House). We spoke with Dr. Perlmutter about his recommended brain-health protocol, which uses nutritional supplements to boost the brain's natural ability to protect itself. Beginning right now, you can start to improve the long-term health of your brain simply by using certain nutrients, many of which already may be familiar to you…

HOW NRF2 WORKS

Functioning inside the individual cells of the brain, Nrf2 helps to produce billions of brain-protective antioxidant molecules—far more than you could consume in oral supplements. One of the brain antioxidants that it produces —Glutathione. You may have heard about this antioxidant and its ability to eliminate free radicals. Most people don't have enough glutathione in their bodies—especially since glutathione can become depleted because of illness and aging.

As it turns out, glutathione is especially effective at protecting the brain. It destroys free radicals and removes toxins from the brain, and it regenerates other antioxidants, such as vitamin C, which also destroy free radicals.

Glutathione also has been shown to prevent ALS in lab animals, and Italian researchers have reported significant improvements in Parkinson's patients who received intravenous glutathione. Conversely, low levels of glutathione have been linked to increased incidence of Alzheimer's, Parkinson's and ALS in studies with humans.

MAXIMIZING YOUR NRF2

When patients are treated for these neurodegenerative diseases, they are given drugs that treat the symptoms, not the disease itself. But by activating Nrf2, we can directly tackle the inflammation and oxidative stress that affect the brain.

I have adapted Dr. Perlmutter's protocol for brain health in my own practice. I recommend it for patients who already have neuro-degenerative conditions, such as Parkinson's or ALS. I also recommend it for patients with dementia…Alzheimer's…and (starting at about age 40) for those who have a family history of these conditions (two or more family members with either dementia or Alzheimer's) as a way to boost brain health and protect the brain.

I have patients take these supplements based on their conditions. Those with neurodegenerative conditions generally take all of the supplements described below, while those who want to prevent these illnesses can take several of these nutrients.

• **N-acetylcysteine (NAC) and alpha-lipoic acid (ALA).** These two natural substances can boost glutathione which, in turn, triggers Nrf2. I recommend that patients take the antioxidants NAC (500 mg to 1,000 mg daily) and ALA (100 mg to 300 mg daily). ALA can reduce blood glucose, so patients with diabetes need to be monitored. For more details about boosting glutathione, go to *www.bottomlinepublications.com* (search "boost glutathione").

Other nutrients that activate Nrf2 include the following. Note that you can't get the therapeutic benefit of these nutrients by eating foods containing these nutrients.

• **Docosahexaenoic acid (DHA).** More than two-thirds of the dry weight of the human brain is fat, and one-quarter of that fat consists of the omega-3 fatty acid DHA, which is found in fish oil and krill oil. Studies have shown that DHA can help with memory problems.

Not only does DHA dramatically boost Nrf2-related antioxidant activity, it also increases production of brain-derived neurotrophic factor (BDNF). BDNF is a protein that stimulates the growth of new neurons and synapses and helps protect neurons against damage from trauma (such as a bump on the head or temporary lack of oxygen, as in a stroke), environmental toxins and the stress hormone cortisol. Studies have linked low levels of BDNF to increased incidence of Alzheimer's, epilepsy, anorexia nervosa, depression, schizophrenia and obsessive-compulsive disorder.

Dose: 1,000 mg daily. DHA has a blood-thinning effect, so if you take blood-thinning medication, check with your doctor before taking DHA. If you already take an omega-3 supplement, check the amounts of DHA and EPA in your supplement. If you need more DHA to reach 1,000 mg, look for a product that offers DHA only.

• **Curcumin.** This nutrient, the active ingredient in the Indian spice turmeric, has a powerful stimulating effect on Nrf2. Like DHA, it also has powerful anti-inflammatory benefits and increases the brain's production of BDNF.

Dose: 200 mg to 400 mg of turmeric extract containing 95% curcuminoids daily.

• **Sulforaphane.** The active ingredient in broccoli and one of the most potent activators of Nrf2, sulforaphane is available in supplement form. It stimulates liver enzymes that clear carcinogenic metabolites from the body and brain.

Dose: 200 mg to 500 mg of broccoli seed extract daily.

• **Pterostilbene.** This chemical gives blueberries their powerful antioxidant effects. It's chemically related to the more familiar and popular supplement resveratrol but appears to be utilized more readily by the body, and it is especially effective at boosting glutathione production.

Dose: 50 mg to 100 mg daily of pterostilbene. Don't use this supplement if you are allergic to berries.

• **Green tea extract.** Antioxidants in green tea improve brain health because they eliminate free radicals. Other compounds in green tea help the body neutralize and eliminate environmental and dietary toxins. This potent antioxidant also works in part by stimulating Nrf2.

Dose: 200 mg to 400 mg daily of green tea extract.

• **Nrf2 Activator.** For patients who would rather have the convenience of taking just one supplement (instead of the several described above), I recommend Nrf2 Activator. Developed by Dr. Perlmutter, it activates Nrf2 in the body with many of the nutrients listed above, including curcumin, sulforaphane, pterostilbene and green tea extract. The supplement is manufactured by Xymogen, a company for which Dr. Perlmutter is chairman of the medical board of advisers and chief neuroscience officer (and in which he has a financial interest). Nrf2 Activator is available only through health professionals. Have your physician contact Xymogen (800-647-6100, *www.xymogen.com*).

REPORT #59
Listen Up! These Vitamins Can Prevent Hearing Loss

Josef M. Miller, PhD, professor of otolaryngology at University of Michigan Medical School, Ann Arbor, and Karolinska Institute in Stockholm. He is director of the Cochlear Signaling and Tissue Engineering Laboratory at Kresge Hearing Research Institute, also in Ann Arbor.

If you're middle-aged or older, you've probably heard about—or experienced for yourself—"age-related" hearing loss. Many people do lose some of their hearing with advancing age. That's the bad news.

The good news is that recent research has shown that much of this hearing loss can be prevented with certain nutrients. The right foods and supplements actually can help you hear better.

SILENT DAMAGE

Exposure to loud noises over a lifetime is a major cause of *presbycusis*, hearing loss that is associated with age and heredity. A structure in the inner ear called the *cochlea* is lined with thousands of tiny hairs that translate sound vibrations into electrical signals. Noise can damage these hairs and, over time, may result in hearing loss.

Why this happens: Loud noises trigger the production of free radicals, molecules produced in the inner ear that damage the cochlear hairs. Prolonged exposure to noise also causes a constriction of blood vessels and reduces circulation to the inner ear.

In laboratory studies at the University of Michigan, animals were exposed to sounds measuring 120 decibels, about the volume of a rock concert.

During this research, some animals were given the antioxidant-rich nutrients magnesium, beta-carotene (the body converts beta-carotene to vitamin A) and vitamins C and E one hour prior to the noise exposure and then once daily for five days. The test animals had 75% to 80% less hearing loss than animals given their normal food.

WHY NUTRITION HELPS

The antioxidants in fruits, vegetables, whole grains and other plant foods help fight free radicals and inflammation throughout the body, including in the inner ear. People who consume a lot of these nutrients on a regular basis get the most protection because free radical damage persists even when the noise is gone.

The largest spike in free radicals occurs while the noise is present. After that, free radicals intermittently decline and spike again. This cycle continues for five to seven days after the initial exposure, probably because free radicals are produced by the body as it attempts to heal noise-related damage within the inner ear. *Recommended nutrients...*

BEST COMBO

Taken together, the combination of nutrients beta-carotene, magnesium and vitamins C and E seems to be most effective at preventing cell damage. Each one inhibits the formation of free radicals in cells in different parts of the body. Vitamin E and beta-carotene reduce free radicals that are formed in the lipid (fatty) portions of cells, while vitamin C acts in the watery compartments. Magnesium dilates blood vessels, improves inner-ear circulation and prevents a noise-induced reduction in blood flow followed by a rebound increase (which would lead to an additional increase in free radicals).

Recommended doses: 18 milligrams (mg) beta-carotene...500 mg vitamin C...267 mg vitamin E (in the form of alpha-tocopherol)... and 312 mg magnesium. These doses are the equivalents of those used in the studies and are only slightly different from the minimum recommended levels.

Studies have shown that the best time to take nutritional supplements to protect your hearing is about 24 hours before an anticipated noise exposure, such as a concert or a car race.

When you're exposed to loud noises that you didn't anticipate, you can gain protection by increasing your antioxidant intake afterward. Antioxidants have been shown to reduce noise damage in animals when taken as much as three days following noise exposure—although protection was greater when taken one day after the noise.

FOLATE

The Blue Mountains Hearing Study (a survey of age-related hearing loss) collected data on dietary habits and measured levels of hearing loss in nearly 3,000 participants. Those with the lowest blood levels of folate were 39% more likely to experience hearing loss than those with the highest levels. Folate—the supplemental form is folic acid—is an antioxidant that also lowers levels of *homocysteine*, an amino acid that indicates the presence of inflammation in the body. Reducing homocysteine with folate or folic acid may reduce inflammatory damage and possibly improve circulation to the inner ear.

Recommended dose: I advise patients to get 400 micrograms (mcg) daily. You can get this much in one or two servings of many fortified breakfast cereals. Most multinutrient supplements also include folic acid. Foods rich in folate include spinach (100 mcg in one-half cup cooked) and asparagus (85 mcg in four spears).

OMEGA-3 FATTY ACIDS

In the Blue Mountains Hearing Study, those who ate fish two or more times a week were 42% less likely to suffer from age-related hearing loss than those who ate less than one weekly serving of fish.

Recommended: The omega-3 fatty acids in fish are among the healthiest nutrients you can eat. Two or more fish servings a week are probably ideal.

ZINC

This mineral is a chelator that binds to iron and helps remove it from the body. This process is important for hearing because iron plays a role in the formation of free radicals.

Recommended dose: The recommended daily allowance (RDA) is 11 mg zinc for men and 8 mg for women. A serving of beef can supply nearly 9 mg of zinc. Oysters, the richest source, provide 76.7 mg in a half-dozen.

REPORT #60
Cancer-Free in a Week

Mark S. Kaminski, MD, professor of internal medicine, division of hematology and oncology, University of Michigan Cancer Center, Ann Arbor.
Marshall Lichtman, MD, retired executive vice president, research and medical programs, The Leukemia & Lymphoma Society, White Plains, New York.
The New England Journal of Medicine

Just one week of radioactive-based therapy put 75% of people who had advanced follicular lymphoma into complete remission.

BACKGROUND

The radioactive-based therapy, known as *131 I-tositumomab*, is currently approved for people who have relapsed after having chemotherapy. Of the patients who use the therapy, 20% to 38% go on to have a complete remission, and 47% to 68% have some kind of response to the treatment. Some 30% of these patients have remissions that last between one and 10 years.

THE STUDY

Given the success of 131 I-tositumomab as a follow-up treatment, Mark S. Kaminski, MD, lead author of the study, and his team decided to test it as an initial treatment on 76 patients who had stage III or stage IV follicular lymphoma. Each participant got two infusions, one week apart.

FIVE RESULTS

Overall, 95% of the patients showed some response, and 75% went into complete remission. Of those who had a complete remission, 77% remained disease-free after five years. The percentage of relapses decreased each year.

"Instead of a 30% complete response rate, we're now up to 75%, and the complete response is very much key in getting a long remission," says Dr. Kaminski, professor of internal medicine in the division of hematology and oncology at the University of Michigan Cancer Center in Ann Arbor.

The duration and ease of the treatment is almost unknown in cancer treatment. Dr. Kaminski notes that he knows of only one other instance where a quick treatment induced a remission—and that was for the rare hairy cell leukemia.

The 131 I-tositumomab contains an antibody tagged with a radioisotope that emits radiation. Scientists believe that when the compound is injected into the bloodstream, the antibody binds to a certain protein on the tumor cells, so the radiation from the radioisotope can kill those cells. The antibody itself can also kill tumor cells, resulting in a lethal one–two punch to the cancer.

While the results achieved with this treatment were similar to those achieved with other therapies, there has been no head-to-head comparison with other treatments.

The results of this trial may push the treatment, currently used after chemotherapy, toward being a first-line treatment, says Dr. Kaminski.

"It hasn't been compared to the best current therapy, so we still don't know what role this agent would play," says Marshall Lichtman, MD, retired executive vice president of research and medical programs at The Leukemia & Lymphoma Society. "Would it be used alone, used initially, used with chemo? It had pretty substantial activity, so one could begin thinking about using it earlier."

The patients in this trial were also younger than the average population, which could skew results. "This may be the very best therapy for a subset of patients and may be a very useful addition to other therapies for other subsets. All of these details have to be worked out," Dr. Lichtman explains.

IMPLICATIONS

Dr. Kaminski is optimistic. "I think this is going to open the door to people feeling more comfortable…and treating patients with this earlier."

"I think it's an important incremental step," Dr. Lichtman says.

STATS

Follicular lymphoma, the second most common form of non-Hodgkin's lymphoma, is diagnosed in approximately 15,000 adults in North America each year, with more than 90% of those diagnoses made when the disease is already in an advanced stage.

For advice, guidance and support from a follicular lymphoma survivor, visit the Web site *www.lymphomasurvival.com*.

REPORT #61
Strawberries Join the Fight Against Cancer

Tong Chen, MD, PhD, assistant professor in medical oncology, The Ohio State University Comprehensive Cancer Center, Columbus.

Strawberries are high on a select list of super-healthy foods that virtually everyone likes. Now comes news that they are much more important to our health than previously thought. A recent study done at The Ohio State University Comprehensive Cancer Center on freeze-dried strawberries found that the berries were extremely effective in slowing the development of precancerous esophageal lesions. Anything that helps the fight against esophageal cancer is very welcome news. Not only have the number of cases been growing, it's also a very deadly cancer.

BERRIES BRING REVERSALS

The research (which was sponsored by the California Strawberry Commission) was done in China, where the incidence of esophageal cancer—the type known as squamous cell carcinoma—is extremely high. Americans more typically suffer from a different type of esophageal cancer, known as *adenocarcinoma*. Lead researcher Tong Chen, MD, PhD, assistant professor in medical oncology at Ohio State, said that strawberries may similarly affect the type of cancer common in the West because they impact some genes common to both types.

In Dr. Chen's study, in which each participant ate about two ounces of freeze-dried strawberries a day, 29 of the 36 participants—about 80%—experienced at least some reversal of lesion progress, with some moderate lesions becoming mild and some mild ones reverting to normal.

Dr. Chen said, "Our study is important because it shows that strawberries may be an alternative to—or may work together with—chemopreventive drugs to help stop esophageal cancer. But we will need to test this in randomized placebo-controlled trials in the future."

BIG POWER IN A LITTLE BERRY

As a cancer fighter, strawberries have a powerful combination of molecular components, said Dr. Chen. They contain antioxidant polyphenols, of course, and also vitamins A, C and E, folic acid, calcium, selenium and zinc. She pointed out that you can buy all of these in supplemental form, but in strawberries there seems to be a synergistic effect among the components that makes them more potent than the individual components are on their own. Freeze-drying the fruit takes it to an even more impressive level as a nutrient powerhouse—this process removes water from the fruit, leaving a much denser nutritional content within. In the case of strawberries, which are 90% water, when freeze-dried, the end product is 10 times more nutritious than the equivalent weight of fresh berries. Freeze-dried strawberries are widely available now in supermarkets and health-food stores.

REPORT #62
The Ultimate Lab Test: Dogs that Sniff Out Colon Cancer

Hideto Sonoda, MD, PhD, surgery department, Postgraduate School of Medicine, Kyushu University, Fukuoka, Japan.
Floriano Marchetti, MD, assistant professor of clinical surgery, director, Colon and Rectal Surgery Residency Program, University of Miami Miller School of Medicine.
Ted Gansler, MD, director of medical content, American Cancer Society.
Gut online

With powers of smell far superior to those of humans, dogs can sniff out buried earthquake victims. They can unearth hidden bombs or drugs. They can also apparently detect colorectal cancer, Japanese researchers suggest.

Researchers from Kyushu University and colleagues report that a specially trained 8-year-old female Labrador retriever named Marine is able to detect colorectal cancer among patients with up to 98% accuracy.

A graduate of the St. Sugar Cancer-Sniffing Dog Training Center in Chiba, Japan, the dog was initially trained for water rescue and could already detect 12 types of cancer in patients' breath samples before she joined the colorectal cancer study, the researchers said.

The goal of the study was to find out whether odor can become an effective tool in colorectal cancer screening, according to lead researcher Hideto Sonoda, MD, PhD, from the department of surgery at the Postgraduate School of Medicine at Kyushu University in Fukuoka.

The report was published in an online edition of the peer-reviewed journal *Gut*.

STUDY DETAILS

For the study, Dr. Sonoda's group collected samples of stool and exhaled breath from 40 patients with colorectal cancer and also from 320 healthy people. "The tests were conducted from November to June, because the dog's concentration tends to decrease during the hot summer season," Dr. Sonoda noted.

The dog was able to distinguish cancerous samples from noncancerous samples in 33 of 36 breath tests and in 37 of 38 stool tests, the researchers found. "Moreover, canine scent judgment even appeared to be highly accurate for early-stage colorectal cancer," Dr. Sonoda said.

In contrast, fecal occult blood screening—a simple, non-invasive test for colon cancer—picks up early-stage disease in only one out of 10 cases, the study noted.

Based on their findings, the researchers say the canine's evaluation of breath samples was accurate 95% of the time and her stool sample evaluation was accurate 98% of the time, compared with colonoscopy, which is the "gold standard" for identifying colon cancer.

In fact, the dog was able to identify cancers even when smokers and people with other stomach problems were included in the test, the researchers noted.

The tests were repeated three times, Dr. Sonoda said. "The results of all tests were correct, thereby suggesting that a specific cancer scent indeed exists," he said.

The researchers also took breath and stool samples from patients with breast, stomach and prostate cancer. "Canine scent judgment yielded correct answers for these cancers as well, suggesting that common scents may exist among various cancer types," Dr. Sonoda said.

While dogs seem to be able to pick-up the "smell" of cancer, using dogs as a screening tool is not the ultimate goal, he said.

Scent ability and concentration vary between different dogs and also with the same dog on different days, Dr. Sonoda pointed out. "Moreover, each dog can only conduct tests for a maximum of 10 years. So it is difficult to introduce canine scent judgment into clinical practice," he said.

For these reasons, it is necessary to identify the cancer-specific organic compounds detected by dogs and to develop an early cancer detection sensor that can be substituted for a dog's judgment, Dr. Sonoda said.

"We hope that the results of the present study will provide encouragement for the development of cancer detection and solving the biological character of cancer using odor material," he said.

EXPERT REACTION

Commenting on the study, Ted Gansler, MD, director of medical content at the American Cancer Society, said that "this study adds to a small number of other published articles showing similar results regarding bladder, lung and breast cancers," and to a recent conference presentation regarding prostate cancer.

"In addition to these studies, there have been several anecdotal reports of patients whose pet dogs seemed attracted to or upset by skin cancers," he added.

Although the idea of dogs recognizing cancer might initially seem difficult for some people to believe, it also seems biologically plausible, Dr. Gansler said.

"We know that trained dogs can distinguish the scent of one person from another person. Dogs can also be trained to recognize very low concentrations of explosives or illegal drugs in the air. Scientists have already identified some of the chemical differences between normal and malignant tissues, so it is not surprising that some dogs can also recognize these differences," he said.

Some might wonder whether it is time to use dogs in the clinic for cancer screening, Dr. Gansler said. "However, much more research will be needed before we can seriously think about dogs assuming roles in cancer screening similar to their current ones in law enforcement," he said.

NEXT STEPS

One limitation is that the dog in this study did not reliably recognize any abnormal scent from precancerous polyps, although it was not specifically trained to do so, Dr. Gansler said. "In contrast, some colon cancer tests such as colonoscopy can accurately recognize these polyps so they can be removed by the doctor in order to prevent colon cancer before it is fully developed."

The next step is to discover the specific chemicals associated with colon cancer, or with other types of cancers, Dr. Gansler said. "Once that is done, scientists will try to develop laboratory tests that detect these chemicals as potential methods for cancer screening."

Another expert, Floriano Marchetti, MD, an assistant professor of clinical surgery and director of the Colon and Rectal Surgery Residency Program at the University of Miami Miller School of Medicine, said that "the direction should be to stimulate research in finding the organic compound that the dog reacts to."

If one could develop a simple screening test, it could be useful in getting more people screened for colon cancer, he said. "In this country, any type of screening for colorectal cancer is in the order of 40% to 45%. Something like this, if it were simple, would be beneficial."

REPORT #63
Melatonin: New Help For Heartburn

Mark A. Stengler, NMD, licensed naturopathic medical doctor in private practice, Stengler Center for Integrative Medicine, Encinitas, California...adjunct associate clinical professor at the National College of Natural Medicine, Portland, Oregon...author of many books, including *The Natural Physician's Healing Therapies* and coauthor of *Prescription for Natural Cures* (both from Bottom Line Books).

We tend to think of melatonin, often called the "sleep hormone," in terms of—you guessed it—sleep. So what does melatonin have to do with your digestion? The answer is a lot, according to new research. It turns out that this hormone, in addition to regulating our sleep/wake cycle, also can help gastroesophageal reflux disease (GERD). This is very good news!

Known for its symptoms of acid reflux or heartburn, GERD is a very common condition that occurs when the lower esophageal sphincter—the valve between the esophagus and the stomach—relaxes at the wrong time, allowing gastric acid to escape from the stomach into the esophagus. The result is pain and a burning sensation in the chest and throat. Over time, the acid exposure from GERD can damage the esophagus, even causing cancer and other serious conditions.

Melatonin as an effective treatment is exciting news because there are many possible dangerous side effects (such as bone fractures and stomach disorders) that can occur with popular medications for GERD—namely, proton-pump inhibitors (PPIs) and H2 receptor antagonists, which work by suppressing stomach acid production. One study even suggests that their long-term use may increase risk for cognitive decline.

THE MELATONIN BREAKTHROUGH

Melatonin is a naturally occurring hormone that is made in various parts of the body. When produced by the brain's pineal gland (which happens whenever you're exposed to darkness), melatonin has a strong influence on circadian rhythms and encourages sleep. It also has many other beneficial effects. Preliminary studies show that it is an effective treatment for migraine, obesity and seasonal affective disorder.

What many people don't know: The gastrointestinal (GI) tract secretes up to 500 times as much melatonin as the pineal gland. Researchers have determined that the hormone plays an important role in the GI system by preventing oxidative stress on GI cells...regulating cholesterol uptake by the intestinal wall...helping to heal damage to the lining of the GI tract...and promoting the secretion of other hormones that aid digestion and elimination. Studies have shown that supplementing with melatonin can help to treat esophageal ulcers, dyspepsia (upset stomach) and irritable bowel syndrome.

Now there is evidence that melatonin supplements also alleviate GERD symptoms.

One possible reason: Melatonin has been found to reduce gastric acid secretion (although not to the degree of PPIs) and to normalize pressure of the lower esophageal sphincter, allowing it to close more effectively.

In one study, published in *Journal of Pineal Research,* GERD patients received a daily supplement of 6 milligrams (mg) of melatonin, along with L-tryptophan, vitamin B-6, folic acid, vitamin B-12, methionine and betaine (the additional nutrients were administered for their anti-inflammatory and analgesic effects). An equal number of subjects were treated with daily 20-mg doses of the PPI *omeprazole.* Remarkably, after 40 days, 100% of the melatonin group reported no noticeable GERD symptoms, compared with just 65% of the omeprazole group.

My advice: I recommend that patients with GERD take 3 mg to 6 mg daily of melatonin 30 minutes before bedtime. I recommend the sublingual form for those who have trouble falling asleep or the time-release form if they tend to wake up during the night. If you have no obvious sleep problems, take a close look at your sleep pattern and determine if you have a tendency to either struggle when falling asleep or wake at night—and take the form accordingly. Melatonin is not recommended for children or for women who are pregnant.

REPORT #64
New Treatment for Cataracts

New cataract treatment uses an infrared laser to "bleach" the age-induced yellowing of the lens. The procedure, now being tested, takes about a half-hour and could eventually be done in mobile clinics. Cataracts now are treated with invasive lens-replacement surgery by a team of eye surgeons. Cataracts are the number-one cause of blindness in the world.

Line Kessel, MD, PhD, ophthalmologist, Glostrup Hospital, University of Copenhagen, Copenhagen, Denmark, and leader of a study published in the online medical journal *PLoS One*.

REPORT #65
Early Morning Colonoscopies Find 27% More Polyps

University of California, Los Angeles, news release

Early morning colonoscopies detect more polyps than colon cancer screenings done later in the day, and the number of polyps found decreases by the hour as the day progresses, a recent study has found.

Removing polyps is believed to reduce the risk of colon cancer by 60% to 90%.

THE STUDY

Researchers from the University of California, Los Angeles, analyzed data on 477 people who had colonoscopies in a one-year span at a Veterans Affairs hospital. Colonoscopies that started at 8:30 a.m. or earlier detected 27% more polyps per patient than colonoscopies performed at a later time, according to the study.

POSSIBLE EXPLANATIONS

The improved rate in the early morning may be due to better bowel preparation the night before, according to the researchers. They also suggested that doctor fatigue might also play a role in declining detection as the day wears on.

IMPLICATIONS

"We may find that setting a cap on the duration of endoscopic work shifts or other types of adjustments may be helpful," said Brennan M.R. Spiegel, MD, director of the UCLA/Veterans Affairs Center for Outcomes Research and Education and a coauthor of the study.

ADVICE

Dr. Spiegel emphasized that colonoscopy is an effective way to screen for colon cancer at any time of the day and said that people should not worry about getting early morning procedures. (In other words, the most important thing to do is to get one.)

"The impact of appointment time for any individual is very, very small," Dr. Spiegel said. "Patients should feel confident that colonoscopy is helpful regardless of time of day and should be more focused on the quality and experience of their doctor rather than the time of their appointment."

The study was published in *Clinical Gastroenterology and Hepatology*.

REPORT #66
The Truth About Life After Prostate Cancer

Arnold Melman, MD, professor of urology at Albert Einstein College of Medicine in New York City, where he also has a private practice. A former president of the Society for the Study of Impotence, he specializes in prostate surgery and the diagnosis and treatment of male sexual dysfunction. He is author, with Rosemary E. Newnham, of *After Prostate Cancer: A What-Comes-Next Guide to a Safe and Informed Recovery* (Oxford University).

Roughly two million American men are now living with prostate cancer or the aftereffects of treatment.

That's largely because the ability to detect and treat prostate cancer has greatly improved.

Now, about 90% of the nearly 250,000 American men who are diagnosed with the disease each year are alive at least 15 years after treatment.

The downside: Surgery and radiation, the main treatments, can cause serious side effects, including erectile dysfunction (ED) and incontinence.

Important recent study: Nearly half of men who had surgery for prostate cancer expected to have a better recovery than they actually did.

WHAT TO REALLY EXPECT

The complications of surgery (which typically involves total removal of the prostate gland) and radiation vary widely, depending on a man's age, the presence of other diseases (such as diabetes) and the specific type of treatment he receives. For example, a 50-year-old who had good erections prior to surgery will probably have them again within a year or two. An older man with a history of health problems won't do as well.

COPING WITH ED

Some of the nerves that control erections are invariably damaged during prostate removal surgery. This occurs even with so-called nerve-sparing procedures that are designed to minimize damage to nerves that supply the penis. In many cases, a man's ability to have erections can return within about 18 months, but there's no guarantee of a full recovery. In fact, recovery varies widely depending on the age and health of the patient—overall, 50% to 60% have permanent ED.

Men who are treated with radiation may retain their ability to have erections initially, but damage to nerves and blood vessels from radiation increases in the weeks and months after treatment.

Even so, prostate cancer survivors and their partners can still have satisfying sex lives (though the man may have a somewhat lower level of performance). *Here's how...*

•**Consider injections.** The average man is unwilling to stick a needle in his penis when he wants to have sex. But I encourage my patients to consider this treatment because it is the most effective—and always the least expensive—approach.

The drugs that are injected, *papaverine*, *prostaglandin* and *phentolamine*, are often combined in one solution. The injection usually produces an almost immediate erection even when a man isn't sexually aroused. The erection can last anywhere from about 10 minutes to four hours, depending on the dose.

The needle is so small that the injections are virtually painless. Once a man learns how to inject himself, he's given a prescription for enough medication to provide at least 50 doses.

Cost per shot: About $3.

Drawbacks: Apart from the fear of injections, the only likely side effect is an erection that lasts too long. This might not sound like a problem, but an overly persistent erection is painful and dangerous, potentially leading to permanent dysfunction. It can be prevented by reducing the dose.

•**Take a pill.** For those patients who are unwilling to try injections, *sildenafil* (Viagra), *vardenafil* (Levitra) and *tadalafil* (Cialis) promote blood flow to the penis when a man is sexually aroused and improve erections in about 60% of prostate cancer survivors who use the medications.

These medications work best in men who are in relatively good physical shape, don't have other serious health problems and have had nerve-sparing surgery or radiation alone. They're least effective in older men or men with low testosterone or complications from diabetes—and usually not effective at all for men who have had total removal of the prostate and surrounding tissue because they may have suffered nerve damage. Viagra, Levitra and Cialis can produce an erection in 30 to 60 minutes, and it typically lasts two to four hours.

Drawbacks: The medications cost $12 to $20 per pill (sometimes covered by insurance) and often cause headaches, dizziness, nasal congestion and other side effects. These drugs can also be dangerous or even deadly when combined with nitroglycerine medications, taken for heart problems.

•**Use a vacuum device.** This can be a good choice for men in long-term relationships who are comfortable "tinkering" before intercourse.

What happens: Just before intercourse, a man places a plastic sheath over his penis. Then, a motor (or a plastic crank, in less expensive models) creates a vacuum inside the sheath, which pulls blood into the penis. Once a man has an erection, he slips a rubber band around the base of the penis to hold the blood in place for 30 minutes.

Cost: $95 to $550, depending on the model.

Important: Use a vacuum device that has FDA approval and is prescribed by a doctor—the devices sold at "adult" stores may lack safety controls and generate too much pressure.

Drawbacks: Some men experience bruising on the penis. Also, many couples find the mechanical aspect of the devices unromantic.

•**Ask your doctor about surgical implants.** Men who can't get an erection any other way or prefer not to use the ED treatments described earlier may opt for a surgical implant.

Main choices: Semirigid, rodlike devices that are implanted in the penis and can be bent, like a pipe cleaner, into the proper position for intercourse...or a hydraulic device, controlled by a small bulb implanted in the scrotum, that pushes fluid into hollow tubes in the penis, causing them to inflate.

Most men who have these devices like them because they don't need pills or injections or require the steps that are necessary to use a vacuum device. As a result, they can have sex whenever they want.

Drawbacks: Postsurgical infection is the main risk. This occurs in about 3% of nondiabetic men. In men with diabetes, the infection rate is about 8%. The devices are expensive but often partially covered by insurance. Out-of-pocket costs are about $5,000 for the semirigid device and $8,000 for the inflatable one.

URINARY INCONTINENCE

Lack of urinary control is the second most common complication of prostate cancer treatments.

Reason: The prostate gland helps control/block the flow of urine. When the gland is removed or damaged, the urinary sphincter (the muscle that controls urine) has to work alone—and often fails. Most men eventually regain bladder control, but this can take two years or more.

Surgery—to implant an artificial sphincter, for example—may be needed if a man accidentally voids or "leaks" large amounts of urine. *My advice...*

•**Expect some leakage.** Most men who are treated with surgery and/or radiation for prostate cancer will experience some degree of stress incontinence—the leakage of a few drops of urine when they cough, sneeze, laugh, etc. It can be embarrassing, but as long as the amounts of urine are small, it's usually nothing to worry about. It will probably improve with time. Some men who have radiation may also have urge incontinence—a strong, sudden need to urinate.

When men are leaking large amounts of urine or when they're so embarrassed that they feel they can't leave the house, over-the-counter pads can help.

•**Do Kegel exercises.** Apart from surgery, this is the most effective way for men to regain bladder control. (Kegel exercises probably won't help men who are leaking large amounts of urine, but it doesn't hurt for these men to try them.) Start doing them every day after a diagnosis—before cancer treatments begin—to prevent future problems.

What to do: First, identify the pelvic-floor muscles. They're the muscles that you contract to hold urine in the bladder—or to stop the flow of urine in midstream.

Several times a day, squeeze the muscles as hard as you can. Hold for about five seconds, then relax. Repeat this sequence a few times. As the muscles get stronger, try to do 20 or more contractions at a time. Do them a few times a day.

REPORT #67
Why I Love Lasers to Zap Fat

Mark A. Stengler, NMD, naturopathic medical doctor and leading authority on the practice of alternative and integrated medicine. Dr. Stengler is author of the *Health Revelations* newsletter, author of *The Natural Physician's Healing Therapies* (Bottom Line Books), founder and medical director of the Stengler Center for Integrative Medicine in Encinitas, California, and adjunct associate clinical professor at the National College of Natural Medicine in Portland, Oregon. *http://markstengler.com*

How can I get rid of this belly fat?" That is the question countless patients ask when they come to my clinic. My answer to that question (as you might expect) is a healthful diet, an exercise program and some hormone balancing. But as I have observed from countless patients, losing weight in these ways is not easy. So before you schedule that tummy tuck or sign up with some gimmicky program that promises to take inches off your abdomen and waist, find out about a new alternative...

It is a low-level laser treatment (LLLT) called Zerona that's used for body contouring. It has been tested and used by physicians since 2008, but has been FDA approved. (There are other LLLT devices made by other companies. Zerona is the one I am most familiar with.) The procedure is performed by holistic physicians, plastic surgeons and some dermatologists.

Are you wondering why I recommend a laser therapy for fat reduction? Because aside from diet and exercise, it is one of the most noninvasive therapies for eliminating fat cells—and I believe that there's nothing wrong with using technology to help make things easier. Zerona does not involve surgery or anesthesia—and there are no wounds and no pain. I recommend it for people who are five pounds to 25 pounds overweight, who really want to lose that fat and who haven't been able to do it.

WHAT IS A LOW-LEVEL LASER?

One of the reasons I like LLLT is that the energy output of the laser is extremely low, only about $1/1,000$ as intense as the lasers used to perform other procedures, such as those to eliminate age spots and skin blemishes. Known as cold laser technology (because it isn't hot and doesn't burn the skin), Zerona involves a focused light that penetrates below the skin, stimulating receptors inside individual cells. In the case of fat cells, the laser emulsifies some of the fat that they contain, allowing it to move into the surrounding extracellular fluid. From there, the liquefied fat is absorbed into the lymph nodes and eventually released as fatty acids into the bloodstream, where it is eliminated as waste. Unlike liposuction, the cosmetic surgical procedure that removes excess fat from the body, LLLT doesn't eliminate fat cells. LLLT patients retain all the fat cells that they started with—the cells simply contain less fat. And the body uses its own detoxification process to rid itself of the contents of the fat cells.

In a study conducted by Erchonia Medical, the manufacturer of the Zerona laser, and published in the peer-reviewed journal *Lasers in Surgery and Medicine*, researchers found that volunteers treated for two weeks with the laser lost about 0.7 inches from each thigh...0.98 inches across the waist...and 1.05 inches across the hips. The weight loss can be long term if patients continue to maintain a healthful diet and exercise program. If they don't, of course, the weight loss is not permanent.

Thomas Barnes, MD, a cosmetic surgeon in Newport Beach, California, who uses Zerona to treat patients, provided more details on how the technique works. Dr. Barnes also serves as a consultant to Santa Barbara Medical Innovations (SBMI), the company that distributes the Zerona laser.

LOSING INCHES OF FAT IN WEEKS

The Zerona device consists of five individual lasers, each mounted on a slowly revolving platform that allows the laser light to reach a relatively large surface area. Because the energy level is low, patients don't feel anything.

Although this approach is designed to reduce the fat content of areas directly exposed to the laser light, Dr. Barnes has found that the laser produces a systemic effect, draining fat from adjacent cells that aren't directly under the laser beams.

Example: A laser pointed at the torso can remove fat around the arms. For this reason, Dr. Barnes takes additional before—and after—measurements of his patients' upper arms, neck and upper abdomen. While results vary, he reports an average circumference reduction of one inch per measurement area.

Patients undergo a 40-minute session every other day for 14 days. This sequence is necessary because pores in fat cells (which are opened by the laser) begin to close after 72 hours. The treatment works best for those who want to lose areas of fat and for those who need motivation to spur on their weight-loss efforts. It is not for obese patients, who usually need to lose several inches of waist circumference.

Dr. Barnes advises patients to drink eight glasses of water and walk for 30 to 60 minutes every day from the start to the end of treatment to help metabolize the released fat.

One of Dr. Barnes' patients, a 50-year-old woman who had been unable to lose fat in her midsection despite ongoing dieting, lost an average of 1.875 inches from her hips, waist, thighs and knees. Another patient, a woman of 35, lost an average of one inch from these areas.

SBMI reports that more than 15,000 patients have been treated with the laser over the last year. The cost for a full treatment regimen of six sessions is about $2,500. It is not covered by insurance.

ADDITIONAL HEALTH BENEFITS

Liposuction carries significant risk for complications (such as bruising, swelling and tissue damage), but LLLT has never been associated with any adverse effects. There also appear to be benefits associated with emptying fatty acids from the fat cells. The study published in *Lasers in Surgery and Medicine* found that those who had LLLT had significant reductions in total cholesterol and triglycerides.

LLLT is available around the country. To find a physician or other health-care provider in your area who offers Zerona treatments, call 866-463-3244 or visit *www.findzerona.com*.

REPORT #68
The Ultimate Natural Weight-Loss Aid

Stephen Bloom, MD, professor of medicine, Hammersmith Hospital, Imperial College, London.
David Cummings, MD, professor of medicine, University of Washington, Seattle.
The New England Journal of Medicine

Injections of a natural protein significantly trimmed a person's urge to eat, a study found. The discovery could lead to effective obesity treatments.

The protein, normally secreted in the intestine, is called *peptide* YY (PYY), and it cuts food intake by sending satiety signals to the brain. Previous research had shown that normal-weight people don't eat as much when injected with PYY prior to a meal. The latest study has found that the effect is equally potent for the obese, cutting short-term food intake by about 30% in both groups.

"We didn't know whether PYY would work," says Stephen Bloom, MD, leader of the study.

"But when we administered PYY, it was fully effective. That is the first step for trying to establish it as a therapy for obesity," he adds.

THE STUDY

Dr. Bloom and his colleagues studied the effects of PYY in 12 fit and 12 obese men and women. The obese subjects had roughly 40% lower levels of the peptide than their slim peers.

Dr. Bloom says the difference explains why obese people have a greater tendency to eat. "They don't have the same level of satiety hormone that thin people have," he says.

Why PYY was so low in the obese study subjects isn't clear. It could reflect prolonged overeating or it could be the cause of the overeating.

David Cummings, MD, an appetite expert at the University of Washington in Seattle, is concerned about touting the results of this study. "Does PYY help you avoid one meal, or is it a regulator of body weight over the long haul?" he asks. Ultimately, Dr. Cummings says, drug treatment for obesity will likely be a cocktail of medicines that target several pathways to appetite regulation.

REPORT #69
The Blood Pressure Pill That's Great for Your Bones

Bruno H. Stricker, PhD, professor, Erasmus University Medical Center, Rotterdam, the Netherlands.

Felicia Cosman, MD, clinical director, National Osteoporosis Foundation, and osteoporosis specialist, Helen Hayes Hospital, Haverstraw, New York.

Annals of Internal Medicine

Thiazide diuretics that control high blood pressure can also reduce age-related bone loss and the resulting fractures, but the protection vanishes once the drugs are stopped, researchers say.

Studies show thiazides slow calcium loss and may be a factor in preventing age-related bone erosion. Now, Dutch investigators have shown that thiazides can reduce the risk of hip fractures.

In a large population of elderly patients, the use of a thiazide medication "offered a substantial protection from hip fracture," says lead researcher Bruno H. Ch. Stricker, PhD, a professor at Erasmus University Medical Center located in Rotterdam.

THE STUDY

The researchers collected data on hip fractures among 7,891 men and women older than age 55.

They classified patients as those who had never used a thiazide, those who had used a thiazide for a short time and those who had used a thiazide for a year or more.

They also looked at individuals who had stopped using a thiazide for a short period and those who had stopped the medication for six months or more.

RISK REDUCED BY HALF

During up to nine years of follow-up study, researchers found that compared with patients who hadn't taken a thiazide diuretic, those who had taken a thiazide for more than one year had about a 50% lower risk of hip fracture.

However, this lower risk disappeared within four months after the medication was stopped, the research team says.

WHAT THE RESEARCH IMPLICATIONS ARE

Because thiazide diuretics are relatively safe, Dr. Stricker believes that they might be useful for treating older patients who have high blood pressure and who are also at risk for hip fracture.

"But I do not advise using thiazides primarily to protect against hip fracture if you do not have hypertension—not until a clinical trial has demonstrated that it is truly effective and how big that effect is," he cautions.

According to Dr. Stricker, based on the current study's findings, "it is reasonable to treat an older woman with hypertension who is also [prone] to hip fracture with a thiazide as a first medication."

FINDINGS SUPPORT OTHER STUDIES

Felicia Cosman, MD, clinical director of the National Osteoporosis Foundation, comments that these findings are consistent with other studies. It is not surprising that the protective effect of thiazide medications wears off after drug use is discontinued. This is a common occurrence with numerous other medications, she explains.

"We still need to follow the same preventive measures for osteoporosis. People need to maximize their calcium and vitamin D intake, exercise regularly and reduce any possible risk factors," she advises.

REPORT #70
Ginger Slows Tumor Growth by 56%

Geovanni Espinosa, ND, director, Integrative Urology Center, NYU Langone Medical Center, New York City. *www.drgeo.com*

Can ginger really help men with prostate cancer? This time-honored remedy is well known for other, less serious problems—including occasional indigestion, muscle soreness, nausea and even arthritis pain. But if ginger can help men manage, or even someday cure, this dangerous cancer, that puts it on another level entirely.

ANTITUMOR BENEFITS WITHOUT TOXIC EFFECTS

There's no doubt that ginger is a nutritional powerhouse—previous research has shown that many of the phytochemicals that make up ginger are packed with anti-inflammatory, antioxidant and antiproliferative powers. Some have been shown, individually, to reduce the risk of developing cancer, and others have been shown to slow tumor growth if cancer occurs. Researchers at Georgia State University in Atlanta studied what effect whole ginger extract might have on prostate cancer, specifically, because other studies have shown that a high intake of fruits and vegetables (which also are high in phytochemicals) help prevent prostate cancer.

After implanting human prostate cancer in mice, investigators fed half of them whole ginger extract (the human equivalent of about 3.5 ounces of fresh ginger) every day for eight weeks, while the other half, the control group, was fed no ginger. *Researchers found…*

- **In the mice that were fed ginger, there was an inhibition (or slowing) of tumor growth by an average of 56%,** compared with no inhibition of tumor growth in the control group that received no ginger.

- **Among the ginger-fed mice, there were no toxic effects in healthy tissue such as the gut or bone marrow.** This is a promising finding, because if these were humans with prostate cancer and they were given a typical treatment of chemotherapy, there would be a high likelihood of toxic side effects, such as neuropathy, nausea, hair loss, mouth sores, diarrhea and permanent infertility.

These findings appeared in the *British Journal of Nutrition*.

AN ANTICANCER DIET

Geovanni Espinosa, ND, director of clinical trials at the Integrative Urology Center at NYU Langone Medical Center in New York City believes that the Georgia State study provides sufficient information to encourage most prostate cancer patients to include ginger in their diets—so talk to your doctor.

And it's easy to do—you can grate it or slice it to mix with vegetables, rice, salad dressings and smoothies. Ginger tea (made from the root) is delicious, and it's easy to brew. Just simmer about and inch or so of ginger slices in water for 10 minutes.

Caution: Dr. Espinosa noted that ginger is not 100% risk-free—for example, in rare cases, high amounts of ginger might worsen a bleeding disorder, reduce blood sugar too much if you're diabetic and interfere with blood pressure drugs and certain heart medications, such as *digoxin* and *digitoxin*. So the possible side effects of extensive treatment with ginger need to be studied in humans.

REPORT #71
Seek Support to Survive Diabetes

Paul Ciechanowski, MD, MPH, associate professor, psychiatry and behavioral sciences, associate director, Psychosomatic Medicine Fellowship, University of Washington School of Medicine, program director, CHAMMP Training Institute, Harborview Medical Center, affiliate investigator, Group Health Research Institute, and CEO/founder, Samepage, Seattle.

Vasudevan A. Raghavan, MBBS, MD, director, cardiometabolic and lipid clinic and medical weight management service, division of endocrinology, Scott & White Healthcare, Temple, Texas.

Diabetes Care

People with diabetes do much better, in terms of survival, if they can turn to others for support in times of need, recent research suggests.

The study found that those who are more independent and feel they don't need help from others have a 33% increased risk of dying over a five-year period.

"These are self-reliant, pull-yourself-up-by-your-bootstraps, self-starters and go-getters. But, in the health-care setting with a chronic illness, what is normally an advantage can become a liability over time," said Paul Ciechanowski, MD, an associate professor in the department of psychiatry and behavioral sciences at the University of Washington School of Medicine.

"Day in, day out, when you have the mortgage to pay, the kids to get to soccer, work deadlines, medications to take and refill, exercise that needs to be done, healthy food that needs to be cooked, and doctors' appointments, it all starts to break down if you're trying to do it all on your own," he said.

BACKGROUND

Previous research has found that people who have chronic illnesses, including diabetes, who lack a good support system are more likely to die, according to background information in the study.

Dr. Ciechanowski and his colleagues wanted to expand on past research and see what effect personality type had on the risk of mortality in the presence of chronic illness.

STUDY DETAILS

The researchers recruited 3,535 non-depressed adults with either type 1 or type 2 diabetes. They found that 53.8% of the study participants had an interactive relationship style, meaning that they had a greater propensity to reach out to others, according to the study. The remainder—46.2%—had an independent relationship style. These people have difficulty reaching out to others and may have a hard time trusting other people, the study found.

The death rate for those in the interactive group was 29 per 1,000 individuals, compared with 39 per 1,000 in the independent group. That means independent people have a 33% increased risk of death, according to the study.

Results of the study were published in *Diabetes Care*.

EXPERT COMMENTARY

"Much of this study is quite intuitive," said Vasudevan Raghavan, MBBS, MD, director of the cardiometabolic and lipid clinic, and the medical weight management service at Scott & White Healthcare in Temple, Texas. "Having a support system provides additional incentive to do the right thing. For example, if you have a mother who visits or calls frequently, she may remind you to get to your doctor's appointment and refill your medication, which prompts you to do it."

Dr. Raghavan said one finding that was particularly telling was that even though people with an interactive style had a higher body mass index (BMI), they still had a lower risk of death. BMI is a measurement of body fatness that takes into account a person's height and weight. Normally, a higher BMI in people with diabetes would tend to be associated with a higher risk of death.

Unfortunately, Dr. Raghavan said, "you can't provide a social prescription. You can't mandate that people reach out to or live with others."

HELPFUL STRATEGIES

Both Dr. Ciechanowski and Dr. Raghavan said these findings should prompt doctors to try to consider a person's relationship style in treatment.

"We need to develop different approaches for people who aren't able to collaborate. Often, they'd love extra help, but are afraid to reach out," said Dr. Ciechanowski. Possible options are e-mails, telephone calls or appointments with other health-care professionals, he said.

REPORT #72
Drop Pounds and Blood Sugar—with Vinegar

Mark A. Stengler, NMD, naturopathic medical doctor and leading authority on the practice of alternative and integrated medicine. Dr. Stengler is author of the *Health Revelations* newsletter, author of *The Natural Physician's Healing Therapies* (Bottom Line Books), founder and medical director of the Stengler Center for Integrative Medicine in Encinitas, California, and adjunct associate clinical professor at the National College of Natural Medicine in Portland, Oregon. *http://markstengler.com*

Vinegar has been used as a folk medicine for such things as headaches and indigestion. Now several studies reinforce its benefit for weight management and blood sugar control. Researchers believe that it is the acetic acid in any type of vinegar (apple cider, balsamic, white or red wine) that produces this effect, interfering with enzymes involved in the digestion of carbohydrates and those that alter glucose metabolism (so that insulin does not spike).

One recent study found that mice fed a high-fat diet—and given acetic acid—developed up to 10% less body fat than those not given acetic acid. Another study found that having small amounts of vinegar at bedtime seemed to reduce waking blood glucose levels in people.

More studies need to be done on vinegar, but it does seem that people can benefit from sprinkling vinegar on salads...adding a teaspoon to marinades...and adding a few drops to mustard. For blood sugar balance (for those with diabetes or on diabetes medication) or weight loss, dilute one to two tablespoons (some people start with teaspoons) in an equal amount of water—and drink it at the beginning of a meal.

REPORT #73
The "Coffee Cure" For High Blood Sugar

Mark A. Pereira, PhD, associate professor of epidemiology and community health, University of Minnesota, Minneapolis.
Rob M. van Dam, PhD, research scientist, Harvard School of Public Health, Boston.
Archives of Internal Medicine

In an 11-year study, drinking coffee cut women's risk of developing diabetes. The greatest reduction was seen in those who drank decaffeinated coffee, said researchers.

THE STUDY

In the study, researchers gathered data on nearly 29,000 older women who answered questions about their risk factors for diabetes, such as age, body mass index (BMI), physical activity and smoking. They also reported on their consumption of various foods and beverages, including regular and decaffeinated coffee.

Adjusting for these risk factors, the researchers found that women who drank more than six cups of any type of coffee daily were 22% less likely to develop type 2 diabetes compared with those who did not drink coffee.

Diabetes risk dropped even more—by 33%—for those who drank more than six cups of decaf per day, the study authors found.

THE ANTIOXIDANT EFFECT

"In our study, for whatever reason, it doesn't look like caffeine has anything to do with [the reduction in diabetes risk]," said lead researcher Mark A. Pereira, PhD, an associate professor of epidemiology and community health at the University of Minnesota, Minneapolis.

Dr. Pereira pointed out that coffee includes many powerful antioxidant chemicals similar to those found in berries and grapes. "When you get up to four or five or more cups per day, you might have very powerful antioxidant activity," he said.

Rob M. van Dam, PhD, part of a research team in the Netherlands that first reported the protective effect of coffee, was not surprised by the results of this study. "People think that if coffee causes it, it must be the caffeine. But coffee is a very complex mixture," he said.

SLOWING DOWN SUGAR ABSORPTION

One component of coffee, chlorogenic acid, seems to be able to slow the absorption of sugar by cells. Studies in rats found that this molecule lowered blood-sugar levels, said Dr. van Dam.

In addition to coffee, chlorogenic acid is abundant in both red wine and chocolate.

"People think that nutritionists are always recommending things they don't like, but that's not true," Dr. van Dam said.

Still, Dr. van Dam and Dr. Pereira agreed that it was too early to single out any one component of coffee as beneficial.

"Clearly, the next step is experimental studies in humans," Dr. van Dam said.

REPORT #74
Diabetes Reversed!

Annals of Surgery
University of Pittsburgh Medical Center news release

The weight-loss procedure called gastric bypass surgery, which has been gaining popularity recently, can improve or eliminate type 2 diabetes in people who are obese, according to Pennsylvania researchers.

Laparoscopic gastric bypass surgery makes the stomach smaller. Patients lose weight because a smaller stomach can't take in as much food.

THE STUDY

A study by scientists at the University of Pittsburgh Medical Center found that 83% of obese patients with type 2 diabetes who underwent the operation saw improvement in, and even total reversal of, their disease.

"Most patients in the study with type 2 diabetes who underwent bypass surgery achieved excellent biochemical [blood sugar] control and were able to reap the clinical benefits of withdrawing from most, if not all, antidiabetes medications, including insulin," said principal investigator Philip Schauer, MD, currently director of the Bariatric and Metabolic Institute at the Cleveland Clinic.

"Younger diabetes patients with less severe disease stand to gain more from the surgery by circumventing years of progressive, debilitating disease," Dr. Schauer added.

THE PROCEDURE

Gastric bypass surgery is intended for the eight million or so Americans who are considered morbidly obese—100 pounds or more above their ideal weight.

Morbid obesity is believed to cut between 15 and 20 years off a person's life, according to the University of Arkansas for Medical Sciences.

Most people who have gastric bypass surgery lose approximately two-thirds of their excess body weight during the first year after the procedure. Most are able to keep that weight off for years.

SYMPTOMS

Type 2 diabetes has symptoms similar to type 1, including frequent urination, excessive thirst and hunger, dramatic weight loss (without dieting), irritability, weakness and fatigue, and nausea and vomiting. Other symptoms include recurring or hard-to-heal skin lesions, gum or bladder infections, blurred vision, tingling or numbness in hands or feet and itchy skin.

Symptoms for type 2 diabetes occur gradually over a period of months or even years. Some people who have type 2 diabetes have symptoms that are so mild, they go undiagnosed.

TREATMENTS

There are a number of different treatments for people who have type 2 diabetes, including drugs other than insulin.

Often patients can control their sugar levels through a diet that is recommended by a physician. Exercise and daily monitoring of their blood sugar levels also help.

The National Diabetes Education Program lists four steps to control diabetes on its Web site at *www.ndep.nih.gov*.

REPORT #75
Attention Women: Diabetes Linked to Irregular Heartbeat Risk

Diabetes raises irregular heartbeat risk in women.

Recent finding: When 34,744 adults were followed for an average of 7.2 years, women with diabetes were 26% more likely to develop atrial fibrillation (irregular heartbeat) than women without diabetes. No such association was found in men, but past research has shown an increased risk for heart disease in general in both men and women with diabetes.

If you have diabetes: Ask your doctor to closely monitor your cardiovascular health.

Gregory A. Nichols, PhD, investigator, Kaiser Permanente Center for Health Research, Portland, Oregon.

REPORT #76
Pain Relievers Are Linked to Erectile Dysfunction

In a recent study, men who regularly used nonsteroidal anti-inflammatory drugs (NSAIDs), such as aspirin or *ibuprofen*, were about 40% more likely to have ED than other men. The reason for the link is unknown.

Caution: If you use an NSAID for heart protection or other benefits, do not stop taking it without first consulting your physician.

Steven J. Jacobsen, MD, PhD, director of research at Kaiser Permanente Southern California, Pasadena, and senior author of a study of 80,966 men, published in *Journal of Urology.*

REPORT #77
How to Firm Up Man Breasts

Larger-than-normal breasts can be an embarrassment for older men. All men possess breast tissue and some, due to increasing body fat and/or hormones, experience tissue growth in this area. After seeing your doctor to rule out less common causes, such as kidney failure, overactive thyroid or other underlying medical conditions, tackle the excessive fat—the most likely culprit.

Recommended: Most days of the week, perform 30 minutes of calorie-burning interval training, which boosts metabolism for hours.

To interval train: While jogging, spinning or using an elliptical machine, alternate one minute of heavier exertion with two minutes of moderate exertion. Do this for the entire workout. Add push-ups and bench presses (10 repetitions of each, three times a week) to develop chest muscles and fill out your chest area with nonfat tissue. Results may start to appear in four weeks. Meanwhile, try wearing a swim shirt and get back in the pool.

Michele Olson, PhD, professor of physical education and exercise science, Auburn Montgomery University, Alabama.

REPORT #78
The Secret Cause of Asthma?

R. Graham Barr, MD, DrPH, assistant professor of medicine and epidemiology, Columbia University, New York City.
Susan Redline, MD, professor of pediatrics, Rainbow Babies & Children's Hospital, Cleveland.
American Journal of Respiratory and Critical Care Medicine

Frequent use of the popular painkiller *acetaminophen* may increase a person's risk for developing asthma, a study says.

But experts caution that it's far too early to tell consumers to avoid it.

Women who were taking acetaminophen at least 15 days a month for six years had a 63% higher risk of developing asthma compared with women who didn't use the analgesic, according to researchers.

Reactions to pain relievers can vary. "We aren't trying to say that all asthmatics should stop using acetaminophen," says study author R. Graham Barr, MD, DrPH, associate professor of medicine and epidemiology at Columbia University.

Soaring rates of asthma across the United States have alarmed public health officials and puzzled asthma experts.

Scientists estimate that in the past 30 years, asthma cases approximately doubled in younger children, says Susan Redline, MD, an asthma expert at Rainbow Babies and Children's Hospital in Cleveland. However, the exact cause of this steep climb remains unclear.

Rising rates of obesity—which can impair lung function—have been cited by experts as a possible culprit, as have indoor pollutants, such as dust mites and mold.

But the upswing in new asthma cases also coincided with the increasing popularity of over-the-counter acetaminophen, the researchers say. According to the American Medical Association, approximately 200 over-the-counter drugs contain acetaminophen.

THE STUDY

In their study, Dr. Barr and his colleagues examined data from the Nurses Health Study, which included nearly 122,000 adult women. As part of the study, each participant kept a record of her analgesic use, as well as the development of any new medical conditions, including asthma.

Among women who used acetaminophen for more than half of the days in a given month, "there was a significant increase—63%—in the risk of a new diagnosis of asthma," Dr. Barr says.

POSSIBLE EXPLANATION

Scientists know that acetaminophen lowers blood levels of a compound called glutathione. "Glutathione has an antioxidant effect in the body, particularly in the lungs," Dr. Barr explains. When glutathione levels plummet, "that may reduce the antioxidant defenses in the body, increasing the possibility of developing asthma."

However, the study only demonstrates an association between acetaminophen and increased asthma—not a cause-and-effect relationship. Dr. Barr notes that other analgesics such as aspirin, *ibuprofen* and drugs such as *celecoxib* (Celebrex) have also been shown to affect asthmatics in various ways.

"If individuals happen to notice that their asthma gets worse after they take aspirin or nonsteroidals or acetaminophen, it's worth reassessing that usage," Dr. Barr says. "But we're not making any blanket statements."

REPORT #79
The Secret Recipe for Hair Growth

Jane Buckle, RN, PhD, director, RJ Buckle Associates LLC, Hazlet, New Jersey. *www.rjbuckle.com*

When you hear the word "aromatherapy," you probably think of a scented bath or a fragrant candle.

But medical practitioners in the United States and around the world are using distilled oils of aromatic plants medicinally. Essential oils activate the parasympathetic nervous system, causing relaxation, which speeds healing.

AROMATHERAPY IN ACTION

Plant oils can be used in a warm bath...in a "carrier oil"—such as almond or sesame oil—for massage...or in a lotion.

The aromas can be sniffed from a bottle...a cotton ball...or a diffuser—a machine that emits the aroma into the air.

Clinical and scientific studies support the use of aromatherapy as an adjunct to medical care for treating...

•**Anxiety.** Essential oils that were inhaled for three minutes relieved anxiety in men and women, according to research published in the

International Journal of Neuroscience. Use rosemary, Roman chamomile or patchouli.

Typical treatment: Sniff one to three drops when anxious.

Caution: Avoid using rosemary if you have high blood pressure.

- **Bronchitis.** Use spike lavender.

Typical treatment: One drop of spike lavender in a bowl of three cups of boiling water. Drape a towel over your head and inhale the steam. Do this for five minutes, four times a day.

- **Hair loss.** In people with hair loss due to *alopecia areata*, essential oils helped restore hair growth, notes an *Archives of Dermatology* study. A carrier oil contained a mixture of thyme (two drops), rosemary (three drops), lavender (three drops) and cedarwood (two drops).

Typical treatment: Massage the mixture into the scalp for two minutes daily.

- **Headache.** Use peppermint. If pain isn't gone in five minutes, try Roman chamomile or true lavender.

Typical treatment: Five drops in one teaspoon of carrier oil. Apply to temples or sniff.

- **Hot flashes.** Use clary sage, fennel, geranium or rose.

Typical treatment: Ten drops in two cups of water in a spray bottle. Spray on face during hot flash.

- **Insomnia.** Use ylang-ylang, neroli or rose.

Typical treatment: Five drops in a diffuser placed in the bedroom.

- **Low-back pain.** Use lemongrass. If you feel no relief in 20 minutes, try rosemary or spike lavender.

Typical treatment: Five drops in one teaspoon of carrier oil. Apply to the painful area every three hours.

- **Menstrual cramps.** Use geranium.

Typical treatment: Five drops added to one teaspoon of carrier oil. Rub on the lower abdomen and lower back every three hours.

- **Muscle spasms.** Use clary sage, sage or try lavender.

Typical treatment: Five drops added to one teaspoon of carrier oil. Apply to the affected muscles at least every three hours.

- **Osteoarthritis.** Use frankincense, rosemary or true lavender.

Typical treatment: Five drops added to one teaspoon of carrier oil. Apply to the painful area every three hours.

WHAT TO BUY

Aromatherapy is most effective when the essential oils are prepared with no extraneous ingredients. One good manufacturer is Puritan's Pride (*www.puritan.com*). Its products are also available in health food stores.

USING AROMATHERAPY SAFELY

Some essential oils are irritating if applied undiluted. Always dilute with a plain carrier oil (scentless organic vegetable oils such as sunflower or safflower are good choices) before using topically. If skin stings or becomes red, wash with unperfumed soap.

Essential oils are flammable. Store them away from candles, fires, cigarettes and stoves. Don't pour oil on lightbulbs to scent a room.

Caution: Essential oils can be lethal if they are ingested—even in tiny doses. Keep away from children and pets. People with asthma or epilepsy and pregnant women should consult their doctors before using aromatherapy.

REPORT #80
Oregano for Arthritis

James A. Duke, PhD, economic botanist retired from the USDA, where he developed a database on the health benefits of various plants (*http://www.ars-grin.gov/duke*). He is author of numerous books including *The Green Pharmacy Guide to Healing Foods* (Rodale).

Oregano helps alleviate osteoarthritis and other inflammatory conditions, such as rheumatoid arthritis. You might be surprised to learn that this favorite spice of Italian cooking contains natural compounds that have many of the same effects as the powerful anti-inflammatory COX-2 inhibitor drug *celecoxib* (Celebrex).

In addition, oregano contains dozens of other anti-inflammatory compounds that act as muscle relaxants and pain relievers. Unlike celecoxib, which may increase heart attack risk in some people, oregano actually *protects* the heart by helping to prevent blood clots and irregular heart rhythms.

Best uses: Use oregano liberally on salads or on pizzas. Oregano also can be mixed with peppermint and/or spearmint for a hot or iced mixed-herb tea. If you prefer to take an anti-inflammatory supplement, oregano is one of the half dozen spices in a product called Zyflamend (its ingredients also include rosemary and turmeric). The herbs in Zyflamend act synergistically to provide a more powerful effect than each would when used individually. Zyflamend can be purchased in health-food stores and online. Follow label instructions.

REPORT #81
Are Pain Medications Sapping Your Sex Life?

Some pain medications suppress sex hormones. Most men and women taking opioids, such as *codeine*, *hydrocodone* (Vicodin), *morphine* and *oxycodone* (OxyContin, Percocet), show reductions in blood levels of estradiol, testosterone and related hormones.

Among the consequences: Patients may experience loss of libido, depression, decreased energy, mood disturbances, osteoporosis and/or premature menopause. Once the opioid is stopped, hormone levels rebound.

Norman J. Marcus, MD, founder and medical director, Norman Marcus Pain Institute, New York City, and a past president of American Academy of Pain Medicine. He is coauthor, with Jean S. Arbeiter, of *Freedom from Pain* (Fireside).

REPORT #82
The Truth About Garlic—Health Claims That You Can Trust...

Ellen Tattelman, MD, director of the faculty development fellowship at the Residency Program in Social Medicine at Montefiore Medical Center in New York City. She is an assistant professor of family and social medicine at Albert Einstein College of Medicine of Yeshiva University, also in New York City.

Garlic is one of the most exhaustively researched herbs—the National Library of Medicine's Web site lists more than 3,700 studies addressing garlic's effect on everything from elevated cholesterol and various types of cancer to fungal infections.

So why is there still so much confusion about the health benefits of garlic?

Even though garlic has been used medicinally by some cultures for thousands of years, much of the contemporary research on garlic is mixed—some studies show that it has positive effects, while others indicate no significant benefits.

Here's what the research shows...

HEART HEALTH

Over the years, scientists have investigated garlic's ability to reduce cholesterol levels and blood pressure and act as an anticlotting agent to prevent blood platelets from being too sticky—a main cause of heart attack.

Key scientific finding: A recent meta-analysis in China looked at 26 randomized, double-blind, placebo-controlled trials—the "gold standard" in scientific research. In that meta-analysis, researchers concluded that garlic reduces total cholesterol by 5.4% and triglyceride levels by 6.5% compared with a placebo. Garlic powder and aged garlic extract were found to be the most effective at lowering total cholesterol, while garlic oil had a greater effect on lowering triglyceride levels.

When it comes to high blood pressure, some credible research shows that garlic can help lower it.

Important scientific findings: Two meta-analyses showed that garlic reduced systolic (top number) blood pressure by 8 mmHg to 16 mmHg and diastolic (bottom number) blood pressure by 7 mmHg to 9 mmHg in people with high blood pressure.

As for garlic's antiplatelet effect—that is, its ability to make blood less sticky and therefore less prone to clotting—a meta-analysis of 10 trials showed a modest, but significant, decrease in platelet clumping with garlic treatment when compared with placebos in most of the studies.

Bottom line: Garlic does help reduce risk for cardiovascular disease, with positive effects on both total cholesterol and blood pressure. It also has enough of an effect on clotting that I recommend patients discontinue garlic supplements seven to 10 days before surgery because it may prolong bleeding.

My advice: If you have a personal or family history of heart disease, ask your doctor about using garlic (in food or supplements) as part of a heart-healthy lifestyle. Be sure to consult your doctor first if you take a blood pressure or statin drug.

CANCER

Large population studies have shown that people who live in countries where a lot of garlic is eaten—as well as onions and chives—are at lower risk for certain cancers.

Key scientific findings: In China, high intake of garlic and other alliums, including onions, was associated with a reduced risk for esophageal and stomach cancers. Specifically, the study found that people who ate alliums at least once a week had lower incidence of both forms of cancer than people who ate these foods less than once a month.

Meanwhile, the European Prospective Investigation into Cancer and Nutrition, which involves 10 different countries, found that higher intakes of garlic and onions lowered the risk for intestinal cancer.

My advice: If you are concerned about cancer—especially if you have a family history or other risk factors for stomach or esophageal cancer—include one to two cloves of garlic in your diet each day.

INFECTIONS

Historically, garlic has received attention as a potent antibacterial agent. In 1858, Louis Pasteur touted garlic as an antibiotic. Garlic was later used in World War I and World War II as an antiseptic to prevent gangrene.

Bottom line: There have been few contemporary studies looking at the use of garlic to treat infections. However, preliminary research suggests that it may reduce the frequency and duration of colds when taken for prevention and may speed the healing of a fungal infection or wart.

My advice: For most people, garlic is worth trying as a preventive/treatment for these infections (see the following options to take).

SHOULD YOU USE GARLIC?

It's wise to make garlic part of a healthful diet that includes plenty of fruits, vegetables, whole grains and fiber.

Caution: Consuming large quantities of garlic—either in the diet or as a supplement—may cause body odor and/or bad breath. Chewing a sprig of fresh green parsley, mint or cardamom can work as a breath freshener. Hot tea also can help by rinsing away garlic oil still in your mouth. Drinking a glass of milk—full-fat or fat-free—may be effective as well. Garlic, especially on an empty stomach, can cause gastrointestinal upset and flatulence.

Because garlic may also interact with certain prescription drugs, such as *warfarin* (Coumadin), consult your doctor before significantly increasing your intake of the herb if you take any medication or have a chronic medical condition.

Options to consider...

•**Raw garlic.** If you prefer raw garlic, try eating one or two cloves a day. You can chew and swallow it or use it in pesto, guacamole or a salad dressing. Cooked garlic is less powerful medicinally—heat inactivates the enzyme that breaks down alliin, the chemical precursor to allicin.

•**Aged garlic extract (AGE).** If you prefer liquid, AGE is available in this form, which is popular in Europe. Follow label instructions.

• **Powdered garlic supplements.** These are typically sold as capsules or tablets and standardized to contain 1.3% alliin. They usually contain 300 mg.

Typical dose: Two or three capsules or tablets a day.

REPORT #83
You May Not Need a Knee Replacement

David C. Wang, DO, osteopathic physician at The Kaplan Center for Integrative Medicine in McLean, Virginia. A former instructor at Harvard Medical School, he is a nationally recognized expert in treating musculoskeletal pain.

If physical therapy, pain medications and commonly used injections of cortisone or *hyaluronic acid* (Synvisc) no longer relieve your knee pain, don't assume that you need surgery.

Knee replacement is widely known to significantly reduce pain, but 15% of knee-replacement patients still have severe pain several years later. In some cases, scar tissue from the surgery can irritate the surrounding knee structure, which leads to lasting pain.

What's more, the recovery period after knee replacement can be very difficult for some people—for example, it usually takes four to six weeks after the operation before you can drive again, go shopping and do most of your everyday activities. And some knee-replacement patients can never again participate in high-impact sports, such as tennis, jogging or downhill skiing.

Fortunately, there are some highly effective nonsurgical alternatives to knee replacement.

LESS INVASIVE THAN SURGERY

The procedures that show promise for long-term relief are less painful and have a quicker recovery time than knee-replacement surgery. *Nonsurgical approaches…**

*To find a physician with expertise in evaluating and treating musculoskeletal disorders, click on "Find a Doctor" at the Web site of the American Association of Orthopaedic Medicine (*www.aaoMed.org*).

• **Platelet-rich plasma (PRP) therapy.** This is rapidly emerging as one of the most popular remedies for knee pain. It's been successfully used by professional athletes, including the golfer Tiger Woods, to improve healing after a knee injury.

How it's done: A small amount of blood is withdrawn from the patient. The blood is then spun in a centrifuge to concentrate platelets, which are then injected back into the knee to stimulate healing. Injections given in the open space inside a joint are only slightly painful… those given directly into a ligament or tendon typically require a local anesthetic to reduce discomfort. The procedure takes about an hour. Moderate to significant soreness lasts a few days.

How it works: Platelets are small cells in blood that initiate clotting. More importantly, they produce growth factors that stimulate, and accelerate, the body's natural healing process. An injection of PRP stimulates the movement of collagen-producing cells to the injured area. The body uses collagen to repair cartilage and other tissues.

My clinical experience: I've found that about 90% of my patients given PRP treatment for knee osteoarthritis report at least a 50% reduction in knee pain after two to four injections given at four- to eight-week intervals. PRP can heal damaged cartilage, but it won't stop the progression of osteoarthritis. Many patients need a booster shot every couple of years.

Best candidates: PRP can potentially be helpful for anyone with mild-to-severe arthritis who wants to avoid knee-replacement surgery, but seems to work best in younger patients with less severe arthritis.

Typical cost: Each injection ranges from $500 to $1,000. Most patients need at least two injections. PRP usually is not covered by insurance. Risks are minimal but include infection and injury to surrounding tissue.

• **Prolotherapy.** Using sugar (dextrose) injections to treat knee pain sounds like a scam. But this approach, known as prolotherapy, has been extensively researched.

Scientific evidence: In a recent study of arthritis patients published in *Alternative Therapies in Health and Medicine,* patients who received dextrose injections had a 44% decrease in pain, 63% decrease in swelling and 85% fewer episodes of knee buckling after one year.

How it's done: Dextrose solution is injected into the painful area. A topical anesthetic can be used to reduce discomfort from the injections. Most patients get several injections during each session. It takes about 15 minutes. Prolotherapy injections are given every three to six weeks. It usually takes one to three months to notice results, which can last for several years.

How it works: The sugar solution stimulates production of collagen fibers, the body's natural healing response. Sometimes other solutions are used, including sodium morrhuate or phenol.

Best candidates: Most effective for patients with mild-to-moderate knee pain from arthritis or ligament and tendon injury.

Typical cost: $150 to $500 per session. The average patient needs five to seven sessions. It probably won't be covered by insurance. Prolotherapy has a small risk for infection, temporary or permanent nerve irritation or injury, or allergic reaction.

• **Stem cell therapy.** Stem cells are undifferentiated cells that have the ability to turn into specialized cells in different parts of the body. They also have the unique ability to repair damaged tissue by dividing and multiplying almost indefinitely. Stem cell therapy is often used to repair damaged cartilage.

How it's done: Stem cells are "harvested" from the patient, often from fatty tissue or from bone marrow. The cells are spun in a centrifuge to separate stem cells and get a high concentration of them. Patients are given a local anesthetic to reduce discomfort, then the cells are injected into the injured/painful area.

How it works: When stem cells are injected into specific parts of the knee, they transform themselves into chondrocytes, or cells that build cartilage. They can also be transformed into cells known as *fibroblasts* (for soft-tissue repair) or *osteoblasts* (for building bone).

Unlike PRP and prolotherapy, which mobilize the body's repair mechanisms, stem cell therapy directly repairs damaged areas. I've seen arthritis patients with severe bone damage, who I thought would require joint-replacement surgery, improve dramatically enough from this therapy to not need surgery.

Best candidates: People with severe osteo-arthritis who didn't get significant pain relief from PRP or prolotherapy.

Typical cost: About $2,000 to $3,000 per treatment. One treatment might be enough—patients with more severe joint damage may need more. The therapy is not covered by insurance.

REPORT #84
Mike's Miracle Vision Cure

Ione Fine, PhD, research assistant professor, University of Southern California, Los Angeles.
Ivan Schwab, MD, professor of ophthalmology, University of California, Davis, and spokesman, American Academy of Ophthalmology.
Iqbal Ahmad, PhD, associate professor of ophthalmology, University of Nebraska Medical Center, Omaha.
Nature Neuroscience

A chemical accident left Mike May completely blind at the age of three. But his real challenge began when he was finally able to see again.

Forty-three years after May lost his sight, he had an experimental limbal stem cell transplant in his right eye that restored his vision. The procedure is rare, performed on perhaps 100 people each year in the United States.

Now that May, a California businessman, can see, he has found that sight is not that simple. His world consists of colors and abstract forms, not three-dimensional shapes. He can't identify his wife from her face alone, nor can he tell the difference between male and female faces most of the time. Facial expressions remain a mystery.

May's experience represents an opportunity to glean information about how vision works. Scientists knew only that people blind for a long time whose vision returned had difficulties making sense of what they saw. But they didn't know why. Using advanced imaging techniques, researchers now have an idea of the effects of long-term blindness on various parts of the brain.

THE STUDY

Functional magnetic resonance imaging (fMRI) revealed that the parts of May's brain normally responsible for processing faces and objects were inactive. When he was shown something moving, however, that part of his brain showed high levels of activity.

"It's very much a wiring thing," says study author Ione Fine, PhD, who led the project while she was a researcher at the University of California at San Diego. "He can see. He just can't make sense of it."

Because he lost his sight at such a young age, May's brain never "learned" how to see. "Infants just out of the womb see poorly," says Ivan Schwab, MD, professor of ophthalmology at the University of California, Davis, and a spokesman for the American Academy of Ophthalmology. "The brain has to put it all together and the early years are very important."

"You might be able to go ahead and restore vision, but if the brain has not been conditioned to make sense of the information coming from the retina, then it will be very difficult for the patient," says Iqbal Ahmad, PhD, an associate professor of ophthalmology at the University of Nebraska Medical Center in Omaha.

A DIFFERENT LIFE

May says he's better now at guessing what he is seeing than he was when he first got his sight back. He has also become better and faster at figuring out what something is, in large part because he's amassing an internal library of information.

May was a champion skier when he was blind (a guide skied ahead of him and shouted directions), but he had to close his eyes the first time he skied as a sighted person because the experience was so terrifying.

REPORT #85
Natural Painkiller Works Better Than Morphine

Andrew L. Rubman, ND, founder and director, Southbury Clinic for Traditional Medicines, Southbury, Connecticut. *www.southburyclinic.com*

Scientists may have come up with a lead on a new painkiller—a compound derived from an Asian tree bark that appears to alleviate serious pain without causing addiction or serious side effects...which often occur with opium-based painkillers (such as morphine, hydrocodone and oxycodone).

CAN A STICK DO THE TRICK?

At The Scripps Research Institute in Florida, researchers have undertaken a study of *Tabernaemontana divaricata*, also known as crepe jasmine, a tropical flowering plant that has long been used in traditional medicine in China, India and Thailand. Natural practitioners in these countries prescribe various parts of the plant (from flowers to leaves, roots and bark) to heal wounds, fight toothaches and treat skin diseases, fever, pain, scabies and dysentery, notes naturopathic physician Andrew L. Rubman. When it comes to pain, it turns out that one of the most promising elements in crepe jasmine is *conolidine*, an extremely rare constituent of the stem bark of Malayan *T. divaricata*.

In the Scripps laboratory, researchers looked for a way to get sufficient quantities of this hard-to-obtain substance and for the first time created a synthetic conolidine compound. Once they accomplished this feat, they tested its effectiveness on mice. *In various pain models (the researchers used acid to cause pain and inflammation on the paws of the mice), investigators found that the newly synthesized compound...*

• **Was present in high concentrations for up to four hours after administration and passed readily through the blood-brain barrier.** This is important as many areas in the brain are involved in the perception of pain.

• **Effectively relieved acute inflammatory pain in mice.** Scientists measured this by observing such things as how often mice attended to and licked injured paws.

• **Did not show harmful side effects.** Mice demonstrate certain characteristic movements when exposed to morphine—for instance, they become disoriented and walk in circular patterns—which did not happen after conolidine injections.

These findings were published in *Nature Chemistry*.

Researchers are not sure exactly how conolidine relieves pain. It does not bind to opiate receptors in the body and thus is not an opiate like morphine. But it certainly appears to be effective. Much more study is needed, but this may finally turn out to be the alternative to opiates we've been hoping for. Its broad and effective usage over time in India, Thailand and China is yet another reason for hope.

REPORT #86
DMSO—Rub On Quick Pain Relief

Mark A. Stengler, NMD, naturopathic medical doctor in private practice, Encinitas, California...adjunct associate clinical professor at the National College of Natural Medicine, Portland, Oregon...author of *The Natural Physician's Healing Therapies* and coauthor of *Prescription for Natural Cures* (both from Bottom Line Books).

When I am helping patients achieve immediate pain relief for burns, sprains, back pain or arthritis, I often turn to *dimethyl sulfoxide* (DMSO), a remarkable topical alternative medication for pain that has its own remarkable history. *Find out how it can help you...*

THE POWER OF DMSO

DMSO works in several ways. First, as a topical compound, it has analgesic properties and reduces pain quickly—which is why it is great for rubbing on sore muscles and joints. Laboratory studies suggest that it decreases pain by blocking peripheral nerve C fibers. DMSO reduces inflammation by acting as an antioxidant—and so it neutralizes some of the free radicals that promote inflammation. Some evidence suggests that it also can ease swelling, further helping with aches and pains.

Second, DMSO is rich in sulfur—and sulfur is found in every cell and is essential for life. From what we know about DMSO, some of its sulfur is used to create new cells involved in the healing process and in the production of glutathione, the body's most powerful antioxidant.

Third, DMSO dissolves and transports other substances through the skin, which makes it a great carrier and helper in getting other substances into sore or damaged tissues. I have often mixed DMSO with pharmaceutical anti-inflammatory and pain medications, such as *ketoprofen* (Actron) or *gabapentin* (Neurotin), so that people can use these combinations topically without damaging the heart and digestive tract. The best way to mix DMSO with drugs is to have a holistic doctor write a prescription for you and to have it made at a compounding pharmacy.

Used in this way, DMSO can provide real relief of symptoms for many conditions, including back pain, severe arthritis of the hands, shingles, severe nerve pain and many other localized problems. It also has been found to promote the healing of leg and foot ulcers and to speed up healing after surgery.

Where to get DMSO: You can buy DMSO for basic pain relief at health-food stores and online at such Web sites as *www.herbalremedies.com* and Jacob Lab, the Web site of Dr. Stanley Jacob, who helped discover DMSO. (*www.jacoblab.com*). It generally comes in two concentrations, with either 70% or 90% DMSO. Most people find pain relief with the 70% solution. At Jacob Lab, the 70% solution costs $28 for four ounces. This may seem expensive compared with many conventional pain relievers such as NSAIDs, but it works so effectively, has no side effects and is often needed only short-term, so my patients don't mind spending the extra money.

How to use DMSO: Make sure your hands are clean before applying DMSO, especially since it is efficient at transferring substances through the skin. For acute injuries, apply up to four times daily. For chronic conditions, apply twice daily. It can be used for a few days, a few weeks or indefinitely, depending on the condition. Apply a small amount to the painful area and rub it in. Wash your hands after applying DMSO so that excess is not absorbed by your skin.

Within minutes of applying DMSO, many people experience a taste of sulfur or garlic in their mouths that can last for several hours. In general, this is not a big problem. People who are allergic to sulfites can use DMSO. (There is no such thing as an allergy to sulfur.)

REPORT #87
Psoriasis Stopped for Eight Out of 10 Patients

Joel M. Gelfand, MD, assistant professor of dermatology, associate scholar, Center for Clinical Epidemiology and Biostatistics, and medical director, clinical studies unit, department of dermatology, University of Pennsylvania, Philadelphia.

Until recently, there were few effective treatment options for the 1.5 million people who have moderate to severe psoriasis, the skin condition characterized by red, scaly patches.

Now: Drugs known as biologics, made from the proteins of living cells, inhibit the immune cells that trigger psoriasis flare-ups.

Result: Reduced skin-cell buildups and inflammation in patients who have extensive psoriasis—and fewer side effects.

Here's what you should know...

CAUSES

Psoriasis results from genetic abnormalities in the immune system. The disease occurs when immune cells, called T cells, target healthy skin cells rather than pathogens. The attacks trigger the release of *cytokines*, proteins that cause the rapid proliferation of skin cells. Because sunlight protects against flare-ups, psoriasis symptoms often worsen during late fall and early winter.

TOPICAL TREATMENTS

Prescription topical creams and ointments are used when psoriasis affects less than 10% of the skin surface. *They also can be applied to control mild flare-ups...*

•**Steroids are the most effective topical drugs, applied twice daily.** When used long-term, strong steroids can thin the skin, causing stretch marks.

•**Topical retinoid creams,** such as *tazarotene* (Tazorac), usually are used in combination with steroids, allowing for a lower steroid dose to be effective and reducing the risk of side effects. Retinoids can be irritating to the skin.

Warning: Topical or oral retinoids are not recommended for women who are pregnant or planning to become pregnant because they can cause serious birth defects.

•**Vitamin D analogues,** such as *calcipotriene* (Dovonex), are synthetic forms of vitamin D. Typically used along with a steroid, they reduce skin inflammation and slow cell proliferation.

PHOTOTHERAPY

Ultraviolet light (UV) from the sun or artificial sources can slow cell proliferation and reduce inflammation. Light therapy is a good choice for psoriasis that doesn't respond to—or is too extensive for—topical treatment.

•**Narrow-band ultraviolet B (UVB)** phototherapy delivers light wavelengths that treat psoriasis while minimizing the rays that cause burning. Patients usually get three treatments per week. Skin clearing takes at least four to eight weeks.

Narrow-band light therapy can result in total skin clearing in some cases, but skin lesions typically return approximately four to 12 weeks after the treatments are discontinued.

•*Psoralen* **UVA (PUVA)** therapy uses ultraviolet A light and a medication (psoralen) that makes the skin more sensitive to light. PUVA is effective against severe psoriasis, but it's usually a last resort. Patients given PUVA long-term are seven to 10 times more likely to develop squamous-cell carcinoma (cancer of the upper layers of the skin).

• **Combination light therapy.** This particular approach combines UVB light with an oral retinoid, such as *acitretin* (Soriatane). It's effective in 70% to 80% of cases.

SYSTEMIC DRUGS

Patients who do not respond to topical treatments or phototherapy—or whose psoriasis is severe—may need oral drugs such as *methotrexate* (Trexall), *cyclosporine* (Neoral) or acitretin, which suppress the immune system and inhibit rapid cell division. These medications are cheaper than some of the newer psoriasis medications.

Drawback: They have a high risk of serious side effects, including organ damage. However, the damage can be managed if your physician closely monitors you.

Methotrexate can cause liver damage and a reduced white blood cell count. A patient taking methotrexate should have his/her liver biopsied every one to two years to check for liver damage. Cyclosporine can cause high blood pressure, infections and decreased kidney function. Because of the potential for kidney damage, cyclosporine is typically used for only one year. Acitretin, the only oral retinoid approved by the US Food and Drug Administration (FDA) to treat psoriasis, can thin the hair, cause dry skin and lips, cause bone abnormalities and affect liver function. Because of the risk of birth defects, women of childbearing years should not take it.

BIOLOGICS

New treatment options for moderate to severe psoriasis...

• **TNF inhibitors.** Drugs such as *etanercept* (Enbrel) block the action of tumor necrosis factor (TNF), a compound that triggers rapid cell division. *Adalimumab* (Humira) and *infliximab* (Remicade) are approved by the FDA to treat rheumatoid arthritis and more recently psoriasis. Approximately 50% to 80% of patients taking TNF inhibitors experience almost total clearing of their skin.

Drawbacks: TNF inhibitors are given only by injection. Serious side effects aren't common but include an increased risk of infection, lymphoma, neurological problems and exacerbation of heart failure.

• **T-cell inhibitors.** *Alefacept* (Amevive) slows skin cell division by blocking the effects of the T cells. Approximately 20% of patients experience almost total skin clearing.

Drawbacks: Alefacept is given by intramuscular injection in the doctor's office. Side effects may include liver function abnormalities.

For more information, you can contact the National Psoriasis Foundation, 800-723-9166, *www.psoriasis.org*.

REPORT #88
How to Avoid the NEW Medicare Scam

Steven Podnos, MD, CFP, principal, Wealth Care, LLC, Merritt Island, Florida. Dr. Podnos, a practicing specialist in respiratory medicine and a fee-only financial planner, is author of *Building and Preserving Your Wealth, A Practical Guide for Affluent Investors* (Oak Hill).

Nearly 50 million people are enrolled in Medicare, the federal health insurance program for seniors. Generally, it's available to Americans age 65 and older.

Most participants choose "original" Medicare (the term used by the government). They can select any doctor or hospital that accepts Medicare and Medicare picks up most of the cost.

Alternative: Nearly 10 million Medicare beneficiaries—about one in four—have opted out of the original Medicare program.

These seniors have so-called private Medicare coverage, run by companies, not by the federal government. Several forms of private Medicare are available, collectively known by the government as Medicare Advantage programs. *Why people choose private Medicare...*

• **Medicare Advantage programs** may be less costly than original Medicare.

• **Greater variety of comprehensive services are offered.**

• **Participants in original Medicare** sometimes have to pay considerable out-of-pocket expenses. Private Medicare can help you avoid this.

Example: Under original Medicare, you typically pay 20% of doctors' bills while Medicare pays 80%. Your share might be thousands of dollars a year. Many original Medicare beneficiaries buy a Medicare supplement ("Medigap") insurance policy to cover these potential expenses. However, the premiums for such policies can be substantial.

• **With private Medicare Advantage plans, there is no need to buy a Medigap policy.** You can get comprehensive care, often at a lower out-of-pocket cost.

But there are trade-offs. Before making any decisions, it's vital to understand the fine print.

TYPES OF PRIVATE MEDICARE

Most Medicare Advantage programs are health maintenance organizations (HMOs) or preferred provider organizations (PPOs).

Many Americans become familiar with HMOs and PPOs during their working years. A network of doctors and hospitals is offered to covered individuals, who bear little or no cost beyond their premiums if they stay within that network. Generally, PPOs are more expensive than HMOs but offer more coverage for out-of-network care than HMOs.

Downside: You have less freedom to choose providers than with original Medicare.

Until recently, yet another private option—Medicare private fee-for-service (PFFS) plans—was stealing the spotlight from Medicare HMOs and PPOs. According to the Kaiser Family Foundation, enrollment in Medicare PFFS plans grew from 200,000 in late 2005 to 2.45 million in December 2009. But enrollment fell to 1.5 million in 2010 as providers reduced the number of plans offered.

Why they grew: These plans claim to offer the advantages of Medicare HMOs and Medicare PPOs (comprehensive care with, potentially, lower costs than original Medicare) without the restrictions of staying in a provider network.

How they work: If you're in a PFFS plan, you may see any doctor or go to any hospital that accepts the plan terms. You show a card to prove that you are in the plan. But it is up to the doctor or hospital to decide whether to treat you—they decide on a case-by-case basis.

Trap: Some seniors have signed up for PFFS plans, only to discover that many physicians won't treat them.

My advice: Do not use a PFFS plan. They are poorly designed. Just the fact that you may be denied care by any doctor at any visit makes them a poor choice.

HOW TO CHOOSE

When deciding among Medicare options, the key is comparing what you'll pay and get with original Medicare with what you'll pay and get with a selection of private Medicare plans.

Reality: You can never know with absolute certainty whether original or private Medicare will turn out to be the best deal for you, because you cannot perfectly predict your own future health needs. But, in general, the more health care that people need, the more they will benefit financially from using a private network, because their out-of-pocket costs (copayments, etc.) will probably be lower than with Medicare.

Typical costs: Although each Medicare HMO and Medicare PPO has its own rules and costs, participants in both types must be enrolled in Medicare Part A (hospital coverage) and Part B (coverage for doctors' visits). For the vast majority of people, those who have worked and paid Medicare taxes for at least 40 quarters in their lifetimes, there is no monthly premium for Part A. In 2013, the monthly Part B premium ranges from $104.90 to $335.70, depending on the participant's income.

Some private plans do not charge anything more, but many others do...

• **Average Medicare Advantage premiums for 2013 are about $51 a month,** over and above the Part B premium, according to the Kaiser Family Foundation. This includes plans that do not offer prescription drug benefits.

• **Medicare HMOs that offer a prescription drug benefit charge an average of $33**

a month, over and above the Part B premium, according to the Kaiser Family Foundation.

• **Medicare PPOs that offer a prescription drug benefit charge $69 above the Part B premium.** Prices vary widely depending on competitive market forces in each region.

In return for paying those extra fees up front, private Medicare participants may realize cost savings overall. *Examples...*

• **You won't need a Medigap policy.** In fact, private Medicare enrollees are prohibited from buying this insurance.

• **Private Medicare plans also may offer checkups,** dental care and vision coverage—so you might avoid having to pay for these services.

• **Copayments may be lower with private Medicare than with original Medicare.**

Bottom line: Some private Medicare plans can be good deals. Others will wind up costing you more than you would pay with a Medicare-Medigap combination.

If you have used an HMO or a PPO during your working years, and you know how these systems work, a Medicare version may be a practical choice because you'll know how to "work the system" to get adequate coverage while enjoying the cost savings. If you would rather not be confined to a network, opt for original Medicare with a Medigap policy.

Best: Check with your current physicians before signing up for any kind of private Medicare. Some of these programs are very limited in terms of participating doctors and hospitals.

• **Read the plan documents closely.** Generally, seniors may move in and out of private Medicare plans during the annual election period, which runs from October 15 to December 7. In addition, you can switch from a Medicare Advantage plan to original Medicare during a new "disenrollment" period that runs from January 1 to February 14.

After you make such a choice, you're usually locked in until the next annual election period. However, seniors who were misled into signing up for a private Medicare plan can change coverage right away.

Safety net: You can choose to drop private coverage and enroll in original Medicare within specific periods, as described above.

WHAT TO DO NEXT

To start comparing and shopping for private Medicare plans, visit the Medicare Web site (*www.medicare.gov*). Click on "Find health & drug plans," lower left-hand column. Enter your state zip code to find details on what's available, with contact data for each plan.

REPORT #89
FDA OKs Valve That Does Not Require Open-Heart Surgery

Gregory Crooke, MD, assistant director, cardiothoracic surgery, Maimonides Medical Center, New York City.
James Slater, MD, director, Cardiac Catheterization Lab, NYU Langone Medical Center, New York City.
US Food and Drug Administration.

The first artificial heart valve that can be implanted without open-heart surgery has been approved by the US Food and Drug Administration.

The Sapien Transcatheter Heart Valve is designed to replace an aortic heart valve damaged by senile aortic valve stenosis, a progressive and age-related illness caused by calcium deposits that cause the valve to narrow.

One expert called the advent of the device "a revolutionary breakthrough" in terms of expanding access for sick or frail patients.

"This new approach to valve replacement is designed for the elderly and the highest risk patients who are inoperable—or nearly inoperable—by conventional criteria," said Gregory Crooke, MD, assistant director of cardiothoracic surgery at Maimonides Medical Center in New York City, which is already offering the device to select patients. "As has been shown in trials, it should greatly improve the survival and quality of life for this cohort of patients," he said.

ABOUT AORTIC STENOSIS

In aortic stenosis, the heart has to work harder to pump sufficient amounts of blood through the narrowed valve opening. This eventually causes the heart to weaken, leading to problems such as fainting, chest pain, heart failure, irregular heart rhythms or cardiac arrest.

More than half of patients with symptoms of senile aortic valve stenosis die within two years. Open-heart surgery to replace the diseased valve can restore blood flow, but the procedure is too dangerous for some patients, the FDA noted in a news release.

HOW THE ARTIFICIAL HEART VALVE WORKS

The new artificial valve—made of cow tissue and polyester supported with a stainless steel mesh—provides an option for these patients. The valve is compressed into the end of a catheter that's inserted into a femoral artery (large artery in the thigh) and threaded to the site of the diseased valve. The artificial valve is then released from the catheter and expanded with a balloon. The valve is immediately functional, according to information in the FDA news release.

STUDY FINDINGS

The FDA's approval of the valve is based on a study of 365 patients with the condition who weren't eligible for open-heart surgery. Half of the patients received the artificial valve while the other patients received alternative treatments, such as one that enlarges the aortic valve opening by stretching it with a balloon.

Patients who received the new valve did have eight times as many vascular and bleeding complications and 2.5 times more strokes than those who did not receive the valve. However, patients who received the valve were also more likely to be living one year after surgery than those who received an alternative treatment—69% versus 50%, respectively, the investigators found.

SIDE EFFECTS

The most common serious side effects associated with the artificial valve and its implantation include death, stroke, perforation of blood vessels or ventricular or valvular structures in the heart, significant bleeding, leaks around the new valve, and damage to the heart's conduction system, which is responsible for a consistent and healthy heart beat.

EXPERT COMMENTARY

"Often these patients are elderly with numerous other medical ailments that make standard aortic valve surgery too risky to perform," said James Slater, MD, director of the Cardiac Catheterization Lab at NYU Langone Medical Center in New York City. "Medical [drug] therapy is generally not effective and the availability of a therapy that is less invasive and traumatic than standard surgery is an important advance," he added.

Dr. Slater also hopes that "further improvements in these devices will decrease the rate of complications and that further investigations will allow this therapy to be available to a wider range of patients with this disease."

California-based Edwards Lifescience, which makes the new valve, says it will continue to evaluate patient outcomes through a national registry.

PATIENT ELIGIBILITY

The FDA approved the Sapien Transcatheter Heart Valve for patients who are not eligible for open-heart surgery, but it is not approved for those who can be treated by open-heart surgery. The agency also said that patients with congenital heart valve abnormalities, masses or an infection in their hearts, or those who cannot tolerate anticoagulation/antiplatelet therapy should not receive the new valve.

The valve's product label says a heart surgeon should be involved in determining if a patient is a suitable candidate for the artificial valve.

For more on heart valve disease, visit the Web site of the US National Heart, Lung, and Blood Institute, *www.nhlbi.nih.gov/health/health-topics/topics/hvd/*.

REPORT #90
New Treatment for Severe Migraines

An implanted device called Genesis uses mild electrical impulses to stimulate the occipital nerves, just beneath the skin at the back of the head, and block pain transmission in the brain stem. Genesis already is in use in the US for chronic back pain and is approved for migraine treatment in Europe. Some US doctors prescribe it for migraine on an off-label basis.

Stephen D. Silberstein, MD, is professor of neurology and director of Jefferson Headache Center, Thomas Jefferson University, Philadelphia, and past president of the American Headache Society.

REPORT #91
Grow Your Own "New" Heart

Andreas M. Zeiher, MD, chairman, division of cardiology, University of Frankfurt, Germany.
William O'Neill, MD, medical director, Center for Structural Heart Disease, Henry Ford Hospital, Detroit.
Circulation

A recent study by German cardiologists has found that infusing a patient's own stem cells into a coronary (heart) artery several days after a heart attack improves the heart's pumping power and speeds healing.

THE STUDY

The study found that the stem cell infusions increased the amount of blood ejected by the left ventricle, the heart's main pumping center, by nearly 20%, decreasing tissue damage by 20%.

The study, by researchers at the University of Frankfurt, included only 28 patients, and the report covers just the first four months of treatment. But the results have been encouraging and have prompted a larger trial, says study author Andreas M. Zeiher, MD.

"We now have a 12-month follow-up, and the improvement is preserved over this time," Dr. Zeiher says. "Not a single patient in the trial developed heart failure."

Heart failure, or a progressive loss of the heart's ability to pump blood, often happens after a heart attack. The American Heart Association estimates that more than 51,500 Americans will die of heart failure this year.

ETHICAL ISSUES AVOIDED

The stem cell treatment used by the Frankfurt scientists avoids the ethical issues of fetal stem therapy because it uses the patients' own adult stem cells—Dr. Zeiher prefers the term "progenitor cells." These are more limited than fetal stem cells, but still valuable for their ability to transform into a variety of cells, including heart muscle cells.

Some of the adult stem cells used in the study were harvested from bone marrow, and others were heart-derived cells. Both were equally effective, Dr. Zeiher says.

The long-term trial in Frankfurt includes 60 patients. Half are receiving an infusion of stem cells; the other half are getting inactive cells.

This randomized, double-blind experiment—meaning neither patients nor doctors know who is getting which treatment—is essential for verifying that the therapy works, Dr. Zeiher explains.

An important part of the long-term trial will be to show that infused stem cells can migrate from an artery into the heart muscle and form new, healthy tissue, according to William O'Neill, MD, medical director, Center for Structural Heart Disease, Henry Ford Hospital, Detroit. "The more likely they are to migrate, the more likely they are to focus on damaged areas, improving heart function," he says.

REPORT #92
Aspirin Works as Well as Warfarin for Heart Failure Patients

Kenneth Ong, MD, cardiologist, The Brooklyn Hospital Center, New York City.

Shunichi Homma, MD, professor of medicine, Columbia University, New York City.

American Stroke Association, news release

A major head-to-head trial finds that aspirin is equally as good as *warfarin* (Coumadin) in preventing stroke and death in heart failure patients. Heart failure patients are at increased risk for blood clots, stroke and death.

The researchers said that, all things being equal, the findings raise questions about the wisdom of routinely using warfarin, which can cause dangerous bleeding.

The findings were presented at the annual meeting of the American Stroke Association in New Orleans.

STUDY DETAILS

The study is the largest and longest of its kind to date and included more than 2,300 patients averaging 61 years of age. All patients had heart failure and a normal heart rhythm, and were followed for up to six years (average 3.5 years).

The patients were randomly assigned to receive either 325 milligrams a day of aspirin, or warfarin doses meant to achieve a pre-specified degree of blood thinning.

Death, ischemic stroke (caused by blockage of an artery carrying blood to the brain) or bleeding inside the brain (intracerebral hemorrhage) occurred in about 8% of the patients taking aspirin and about 7.5% of those taking warfarin. This difference was not found to be statistically significant, the research team said.

Among patients who were followed for more than three years, strokes occurred in 0.72% of those taking warfarin and in 1.36% of those taking aspirin, according to the study. While warfarin users had half the stroke risk of those on aspirin, the overall risk for stroke for patients in either group was considered low.

On the other hand, the researchers found that major bleeding (other than intracerebral hemorrhage) occurred in 0.9% of the patients on aspirin each year, compared with 1.8% of those on warfarin. That was a statistically significant difference, the team said.

"Although there was a warfarin benefit for patients treated for four or more years, overall, warfarin and aspirin were similar," said lead author Shunichi Homma, MD, a professor of medicine at Columbia University in New York City.

CONCLUSION

Given that there is no overall difference between the two treatments, there is no compelling reason to use warfarin, especially considering the bleeding risk, Dr. Homma noted.

EXPERT COMMENTARY

"There has always been a question about whether warfarin or aspirin is better when treating heart failure in patients with normal heart rhythms, so this is a very important study," noted Kenneth Ong, MD, a cardiologist at The Brooklyn Hospital Center in New York City.

"Until now, we considered warfarin a more potent anti-clotting drug than aspirin, though each affects a different mechanism of clotting," he explained. "In the past, the only reason to put heart failure patients on warfarin was in the case of patients with a history of strokes, transient ischemic strokes (TIA or 'mini-stroke') or an irregular heart rhythm. This study confirms current standards of treatment. Aspirin is just as effective as warfarin in the treatment of heart failure, but warfarin is indicated for high-risk patients."

The US Agency for Healthcare Research and Quality has more about blood thinners on its Web site, *www.ahrq.gov/consumer/btpills.htm*.

REPORT #93
Love: Nature's Powerful Painkiller?

Sean Mackey, MD, PhD, chief, pain management division, Stanford University School of Medicine, Palo Alto, California.

Joe Contreras, MD, chair, pain and palliative care, Hackensack University Medical Center, New Jersey.

Anna Ratka, PhD, PharmD, professor and chair, pharmaceutical sciences, Texas A&M Health Science Center Irma Lerma Rangel College of Pharmacy, Kingsville.

PLoS ONE

In a study involving a group of love-struck Stanford University undergrads, researchers discovered that high-octane romantic love might be a natural analgesic.

Love's painkilling effect isn't just that the person is distracted by thoughts of the loved one—although that works, too. Instead, the researchers found that feeling "head-over-heels" activates the same dopamine-oriented centers of the brain that tune in to illicit drugs such as cocaine.

"These pain-relieving systems are linked to reward systems," said Sean Mackey, MD, PhD, senior author of the paper that appeared online in *PLoS One*. "Love engages these deep brain systems that are involved with reward and craving and similar systems involved in addiction."

"This gives us some insight into potential ways of further probing and ultimately translating that into treatment for pain," added Dr. Mackey, who is chief of the pain management division at Stanford University School of Medicine.

STUDY DETAILS

The authors recruited 15 Stanford undergrads who were "wildly, recklessly in love," said Dr. Mackey, adding that the recruitment process took "only days."

"It was the easiest study I've ever recruited for," he said. "Within hours they were all banging on my door, 'Study us! Study us!' When you're in that kind of love, you want the world to know about it."

The besotted seven men and eight women, who were still in the newly smitten phase of their relationships, came to the study with a picture of their beloved.

Researchers flashed the picture of the beloved while inflicting pain with a handheld thermal probe. As a control, participants were asked to name every sport that doesn't involve a ball, a form of distraction, while also activating the probe.

"To our pleasant surprise, both love and distraction reduce pain to an equal amount and that was good because it more fully allowed us to compare them," Dr. Mackey explained.

The pain relief afforded by looking at the picture of the beloved seemed specific to that act—when participants were asked to look at a picture of an equally attractive and familiar acquaintance, their pain levels did not recede.

Functional MRI imaging of the participants' brain also revealed that, "the brain systems involved in distraction are entirely different from those involved in love," Dr. Mackey said. "In distraction, there was a much higher level of the newer corticol systems involved with classic attention and distraction."

On the other hand, "in love, very primitive, reptilian brain systems that are classically involved with the reward systems that motivate our basic drives were involved," he said.

IMPLICATIONS

Although the students in this study were at an age when love is often in the air, Dr. Mackey believes the results would easily translate to older folks.

"This doesn't require you to be an undergraduate at a university to fall head-over-heels in love," he said. "Even older people can do that."

Nor would someone have to be in the initial throes of a love affair to benefit from love's soothing effect.

"This gave me a greater appreciation that, for a patient in chronic pain, being in a loving relationship may actually provide some analgesic benefit," Dr. Mackey said.

EXPERT REACTION

Still, love can be an elusive prospect for many. Joe Contreras, MD, chair of pain and palliative care at Hackensack University Medical Center in New Jersey, believes that distraction might be a more accessible (but often ignored) pain remedy.

Finding ways to distract yourself is "definitely something that is unfortunately underutilized, I believe, because our [medical] system does not incentivize it and insurance companies don't pay for it," he said.

And Anna Ratka, PhD, PharmD, professor and chair of pharmaceutical sciences at Texas A&M Health Science Center's Irma Lerma Rangel College of Pharmacy in Kingsville, inserted a note of caution.

"This is still very far from [being useful clinically]," she said. "In my opinion, this is just another demonstration of the fact that pain is an extremely complex phenomenon and it's heavily dependent on perception, and that is actually very different across people."

REPORT #94
SHINE Helps Fibromyalgia

SHINE stands for Sleep, Hormones, Infections, Nutritional supplements and Exercise—and this approach has led to improvements in 91% of fibromyalgia patients. Patients should get eight to nine hours of sleep a night…be tested for hormone deficiency and treated if necessary…get treated for any symptoms of infections…have nutritional supplementation, such as B-12 and magnesium…and exercise as much as possible.

Also effective: Taking 5,000 milligrams of *ribose* (Corvalen), a nonprescription medical food, twice a day increased energy by an average of 61%.

Jacob Teitelbaum, MD, medical director at Fibromyalgia & Fatigue Centers, Addison, Texas. *www.endfatigue.com*

REPORT #95
Contamination Alert!

Urvashi Rangan, PhD, director of technical policy, Consumers Union, Yonkers, New York, and leader of a study of 382 chickens, published in *Consumer Reports*. *www.consumerreports.org*

Two-thirds of chickens are contaminated with potentially dangerous bacteria. *Campylobacter* was found in 62% of fresh whole broilers…*salmonella* in 14%…and both types in 9%.

Also: Most bacteria were resistant to at least one antibiotic. Findings suggest that most companies' safeguards are inadequate.

Cleanest brand-name chicken: Perdue—56% of Perdue chickens were free of bacteria.

Self-defense: Thaw chicken in a refrigerator, inside its package and on a plate…in a bowl filled with cold water (change water every 30 minutes)…or defrost it on a plate in a microwave. Never thaw it on a counter—even when the chicken's inside is frozen, the outside can provide a breeding ground for bacteria. Cook chicken to at least 165°F.

REPORT #96
Don't Chop Those Carrots!

Cook carrots whole before chopping them to retain their nutrients. Chopping before cooking increases the surface area of carrots, so more of the nutrients, including vitamin C, disappear into the water. Cooking carrots whole also keeps them tasty—80% of people preferred the flavor of carrots cooked whole over the flavor of ones chopped before cooking.

Kirsten Brandt, PhD, senior lecturer, department of food and rural development, School of Agriculture, Newcastle University, UK, and lead researcher of a study reported in *Tufts University Health & Nutrition Letter*.

REPORT #97
Warning: We're No Longer Sweet on Agave

The "natural" sugar alternative—agave syrup—is no healthier than refined sugar. Agave syrup is being touted as healthier than sugar and used in an increasing number of foods and beverages.

But: With 20 calories per teaspoon, it has more calories than table sugar (16 calories per teaspoon). It contains up to 90% fructose, depending on how it is processed—much more fructose than in high-fructose corn syrup.

Agave syrup is marketed as "diabetic friendly," but there are no studies to support that it is safe for people with diabetes. Some studies even suggest that large amounts of fructose can increase diabetes risk and have other harmful effects on the heart and the liver.

UC Berkeley Wellness Letter, 500 Fifth Ave., New York City 10110. www.wellnessletter.com

REPORT #98
Natural Relief for Fibrocystic Breasts

Cindee Gardner, PhD, DHom (doctor of homeopathy), registered and certified homeopathic practitioner, molecular biologist, herbalist and nutritional counselor in private practice in Pittsburgh. www.cindeegardner.com and www.homeohelpline.com

Among the challenges that come with being a woman, having fibrocystic breasts may seem like a minor one. Unless, that is, your breasts often feel achy and tender...you experience significant pain and swelling before your period...and/or your mammogram is too murky to read, requiring you to have further tests to screen for cancer.

Fibrocystic breasts have ropy, dense tissue and lumpy, fluid-filled cysts. Frustratingly, Western medicine doesn't have much to offer other than over-the-counter pain medication and, in cases where a large cyst causes extreme pain, drainage with needle aspiration or surgery—but these won't help prevent further cysts from forming. So, it's a relief to hear that alternative therapies can ease symptoms and even help resolve the root causes that lead to fibrocystic breasts, according to Cindee Gardner, PhD, DHom, a homeopathic practitioner, molecular biologist and herbalist in Pittsburgh.

The following natural therapies have long traditions of use and (unlike drugs and surgical procedures) have no adverse side effects or risks when used as directed, so there's no harm in trying them to see if they relieve your symptoms and/or help prevent future flare-ups. The products mentioned below are available without a prescription at health-food stores and/or online...the treatments can be used alone or together in any combination. *Options...*

•**Homeopathy.** Homeopathic remedies are tailored to address a particular combination of symptoms, so choose whichever one of the following most closely matches your situation. *If...*

•**Your breasts often feel heavy, hard, stony and swollen**—try the homeopathic remedy called *Phytolacca decandra.*

•**Aching and lumpiness worsen before your period and tend to be accompanied by tearful moods**—opt for *Pulsatilla.*

•**Cysts and soreness occur mainly in the left breast**—consider *Calcarea phosphorica.*

•**Symptom flare-ups are accompanied by itching**—use *Silica.*

For moderate pain, Dr. Gardner recommended using a 30x or 30c remedy three times per day as needed, following the directions on the label...for severe pain, use the remedy every 30 minutes as needed, lessening the frequency as symptoms improve.

Important: When using any of the remedies above, avoid drinking strong coffee or inhaling strong scents of mint or camphor (for instance, from mothballs)—these can counteract a remedy's effects.

If a nonprescription remedy doesn't help or you need to use it more than a few days per month, it is best to consult a professional homeopath. As Dr. Gardner noted, there are about 45 different remedies for fibrocystic breasts listed in the Homeopathic Materia Medica (the homeopath's version of the Physician's

Desk Reference)—so identifying the most effective one for you may require expert guidance. To find a practitioner, visit the Web site of the National Center for Homeopathy (*www.homeopathic.org/practitioners*) or The National United Professional Association of Trained Homeopaths (*www.nupath.org*).

•**Breast massage.** This practice relieves fibrocystic breast symptoms and helps prevent flare-ups because it stimulates the endocrine system to balance female hormones, keeps breast tissue from getting overly congested and reduces stagnation in the breast glands and ducts, Dr. Gardner said. She recommended massaging the breasts with a topical product called Vita-Cal with Poke, available from *www.archeusonline.com,* which contains vitamins A, D3 and E and organic cold-pressed oils (sesame, avocado, mango, nut, etc.). This rich cream, which is easily absorbed through the skin, is designed to help break up cysts and relieve lymph stagnation.

At least once a week: Lie down, breathe deeply and relax. With a dab of the cream, massage each breast for five minutes or more, moving outward from the nipple and using circular motions, first in one direction and then the other.

•**Dietary changes.** Many women report that fibrocystic symptoms ease significantly when they avoid caffeine and limit high-fat foods, particularly meat and dairy products, Dr. Gardner noted. It also is helpful to drink plenty of water between meals and to increase intake of high-fiber, high-water-content foods such as fruits and vegetables.

•**Herbal tonic.** Dr. Gardner also recommended an oral product called Cystic Breast Tonic (from *www.archeusonline.com*), which combines extracts from various herbs including burdock, echinacea and poke root. It works by thinning the lymphatic fluid so that it can more effectively remove toxins and by aiding the breakdown of fibrous tissue, she explained. For acute symptom flare-ups, take 30 to 60 drops four times per day as needed, continuing for up to one week…for chronic discomfort, take 40 drops twice daily. If symptoms persist for more than three months, consult a trained herbalist.

Referrals: American Herbalists Guild, *www.americanherbalistsguild.com.*

REPORT #99
Ways to Fight Lingering Shingles Pain

Salim M. Hayek, MD, PhD, chief of the division of pain medicine at University Hospitals Case Medical Center and an associate professor at Case Western Reserve University School of Medicine, both in Cleveland. He is board-certified in pain medicine and anesthesiology.

Women have the unfortunate distinction of being more susceptible than men to the painful skin disease *herpes zoster,* otherwise known as shingles.

Surprising: Though shingles has long been considered a once-in-a-lifetime affliction, a recent Mayo Clinic study revealed that more than 5% of sufferers experienced a second bout within the follow-up period, which averaged eight years…and that recurrences were 60% more likely in women.

Shingles develops when the *varicella-zoster virus*—the same virus that causes chicken pox and then goes into hiding in nerve cells—becomes reactivated at a time when a person's immune function is reduced. Shingles risk rises with age as immunity gradually declines. The virus follows a nerve path that leads out from the spine, traveling around one side of the body and surfacing at nerve endings in the skin. The inflamed nerve becomes extremely painful and the affected skin (which reflects the location of that nerve path) erupts in clusters of fluid-filled blisters that take two to four weeks to crust over and heal.

Bad as shingles can be, an even scarier threat is a complication called *postherpetic neuralgia* (PHN) that develops in about 20% of shingles patients. PHN is characterized by intense nerve pain that lingers for months or years after the blisters themselves have healed. According to Salim M. Hayek, MD, PhD, chief of the division of pain medicine at University Hospitals Case Medical Center in Cleveland, the burning, stabbing sensations of PHN can be so severe that even the feeling of clothing or a breeze against the skin can be unbearable—and PHN sufferers often experience depression, isolation and concentration problems. *Self-defense...*

For prevention: Get vaccinated. The FDA recently lowered the approved age for receiving the shingles vaccine, Zostavax, from 60 to 50. The vaccine reduces shingles risk by an estimated 55% to 70%...and it reduces PHN risk by 67%. Vaccinated people who do develop shingles typically experience milder outbreaks and may be less vulnerable to recurrences than unvaccinated ones.

For a shingles outbreak: The first sign of shingles usually is a tingling, burning or itching sensation on the skin, most often on one side of the torso (though it can develop anywhere). This usually is followed within a few days by a red, blotchy rash that later blisters...some patients also have a headache and fever.

Important: If you have possible symptoms of shingles, see your physician immediately, Dr. Hayek advised—if taken within 72 hours of the onset of the rash, a prescription antiviral drug such as *acyclovir* (Zovirax), *famciclovir* (Famvir) or *valacyclovir* (Valtrex) can lessen the severity of shingles and significantly reduce PHN risk.

For pain relief: If over-the-counter painkillers don't do the job, ask your doctor about taking prescription-strength *ibuprofen, acetaminophen with codeine, tramadol* (Ultram) or other pain medication.

For PHN: There is no cure (except, in some cases, time), but there are ways to manage the persistent pain of PHN, Dr. Hayek said. *These include...*

• **Mindfulness-based stress reduction.** A program developed at the University of Massachusetts Medical School combines yoga, meditation, support groups and individually tailored instruction to improve quality of life for PHN patients and other pain sufferers. Visit *www.umassmed.edu/cfm/stress* for information, then check your local hospitals for similar programs.

• **Topical medications.** These inhibit damaged nerve cells in the skin from sending pain messages to the brain. The prescription skin patch Lidoderm, which contains lidocaine, is applied at home and worn for up to 12 hours per day. The prescription skin patch Qutenza, which contains *capsaicin* (the "hot" substance in chili peppers), is applied at the doctor's office in a one-hour procedure and replaced after three months. Nonprescription topical capsaicin products, such as the ointment Zostrix, may help—but patients should follow instructions carefully and some still may not be able to tolerate the burning sensation when capsaicin is first applied, Dr. Hayek said.

• **Oral medications.** Options include the neuropathic pain drug *pregabalin* (Lyrica)...the anticonvulsant *gabapentin* (Neurontin)...the SNRI antidepressant *duloxetine* (Cymbalta)...a tricyclic antidepressant, such as *amitriptyline* (Elavil)...and opioids, such as *oxycodone* (Oxycontin).

Topical and oral PHN medications can have potentially serious side effects, Dr. Hayek cautioned—so it is important to work closely with your physician when using such drugs to manage PHN pain.

REPORT #100
Rise in Some Head and Neck Cancers Tied to Sexual Activity

Gregory Hartig, MD, professor of otolaryngology—head and neck surgery, University of Wisconsin School of Medicine and Public Health, Madison, Wisconsin.
William Lydiatt, MD, professor and division chief, head and neck surgical oncology, University of Nebraska Medical Center, Omaha.
Amesh A. Adalja, MD, adjunct instructor, division of infectious diseases, University of Pittsburgh Medical Center.
Bert W. O'Malley, Jr., MD, chair of Otorhinolaryngology—Head and Neck Surgery and codirector, Head and Neck Cancer Center, University of Pennsylvania School of Medicine, Philadelphia.
D.J. Verret, MD, clinical assistant professor, University of Texas Southwestern Medical School and facial plastic surgeon, Plano, Texas.
New England Journal of Medicine

There's a worrisome uptick in the incidence of certain head and neck cancers among middle-aged and even younger

Americans, and some experts link the trend to a rise in the popularity of oral sex over the past few decades.

That's because the human papillomavirus (HPV) is a major trigger for these cancers, and HPV can be transmitted through this type of sexual activity.

"It seems like a pretty good link that more sexual activity, particularly oral sex, is associated with increased HPV infection," said Greg Hartig, MD, professor of otolaryngology—head and neck surgery at the University of Wisconsin School of Medicine and Public Health in Madison.

HEAD AND NECK CANCER DROPPING, BUT TONGUE CANCER INCREASING

According to William Lydiatt, MD, professor and chief of head and neck surgical oncology at the University of Nebraska Medical Center in Omaha, the overall incidence of head and neck cancers is dropping, largely because fewer people are smoking (tobacco and drinking are the major traditional risk factors).

But the incidence of cancers of the tonsil and base of the tongue have been going up over the past decades, he said. And those are the ones that are more likely to test positive for HPV.

"It's gotten to the point now where 60% to 70% of all tonsil cancers in the US are HPV-related," Dr. Lydiatt said.

LINK BETWEEN VIRUS AND CANCER

Although the link between HPV and these types of cancers is indisputable, the association with oral sex is strong but a little more speculative, experts say.

A 2007 study in the *New England Journal of Medicine* found that younger people with head and neck cancers who tested positive for oral HPV infection were more likely to have had multiple vaginal and oral sex partners in their lifetime.

In the study, having six or more oral sex partners over a lifetime was associated with a 3.4 times higher risk for oropharyngeal cancer—cancers of the base of the tongue, back of the throat or tonsils. Having 26 or more vaginal-sex partners tripled the risk.

And the association increased as the number of partners—in either category—increased.

The researchers also reported that cancers of the tonsil and base of the tongue have been increasing every year since 1973, and wrote that "widespread oral sex practices among adolescents may be a contributing factor in this increase."

The researchers concluded that in their study, oral sex was "strongly associated" with oropharyngeal cancer, but noted that they could not "rule out transmission through direct mouth-to-mouth contact" such as French kissing.

HPV INFECTION

In 90% of cases of HPV infection in the body, the immune system clears HPV naturally within two years, according to federal health agencies, but in some cases, certain types of HPV can lead to cervical cancer or less common malignancies, such as oropharyngeal cancer. A 2010 Swedish study, in fact, suggested that the rise in oropharyngeal squamous cell cancer in a number of countries "is caused by a slow epidemic of HPV infection-induced [cancers]."

HPV tends to be site specific, explained Amesh A. Adalja, MD, an adjunct instructor in the division of infectious diseases at the University of Pittsburgh Medical Center. In other words, it tends to stay wherever it first enters the body, be it the vagina (which in some cases could lead to cervical cancer), or the mouth and throat.

INCREASE IN SEX?

So does the increase in incidence mean that recent generations are having more sex than their grandparents?

"The general consensus on the street is that because people's [sexual] practices have changed over time, we're seeing an increase in these cancers," said Dr. Hartig. "I don't know why they're having more oral sex [but] the concept of having oral sex is something that seems less obscure to you than it did to your parents or grandparents."

"The thought would be that the Baby Boomers—the 60s and early 70s generation—probably had more freedom in sexual relationships in general, including oral sex," added Bert W. O'Malley, Jr., MD, chair of otorhinolaryngology—head and neck surgery at the University of Pennsylvania.

And at least in terms of oral sex, that appears true for those younger than Boomers.

The US Centers for Disease Control and Prevention (CDC) reports that, in 2002, some 90% of males and 88% of females aged 25 to 44 reported ever having oral sex with a partner of the opposite sex.

Comparable figures from 1992 showed that about three-quarters of men aged 20 to 39 and closer to 70% of women aged 18 to 59 having ever given or received oral sex.

CANCERS ARE EASIER TO TREAT

The silver lining is that the HPV-related head and neck cancers are eminently more treatable than those attributable to smoking or drinking, even though they tend to be diagnosed at a later stage.

"[HPV-related head-and-neck cancers] have been a lot easier to treat. You can use less-intensive radiation," said D.J. Verret, MD, clinical assistant professor at the University of Texas Southwestern Medical School and a facial plastic surgeon in Plano, Texas.

About 85% of non-smoking people with HPV-positive tumors survive. That number drops to 45% or 50% in people who smoke and are HPV-negative, Dr. Lydiatt said.

And tongue and tonsil cancers remain relatively rare in the United States. The other good news—at least for the younger set—is that there is a relatively new vaccine to prevent HPV infection. It's not going to help those who are already infected, but it "absolutely" could help those who aren't yet infected with the ubiquitous virus, Dr. Verret said.

Meanwhile, people, especially younger people, need to realize that smoking is not the only risk factor for head and neck cancer. If you find a lump in your neck, even if you're only 20 or 30, "pay attention to it," Dr. Lydiatt said.